# The
# Simple
# Diet

# The Simple Diet

## A DOCTOR'S SCIENCE-BASED PLAN

JAMES W. ANDERSON, M.D.,
AND NANCY J. GUSTAFSON, M.S., R.D.

BERKLEY BOOKS, NEW YORK

**THE BERKLEY PUBLISHING GROUP**
**Published by the Penguin Group**
**Penguin Group (USA) Inc.**
**375 Hudson Street, New York, New York 10014, USA**
Penguin Group (Canada), 90 Eglinton Avenue East, Suite 700, Toronto, Ontario M4P 2Y3, Canada
(a division of Pearson Penguin Canada Inc.)
Penguin Books Ltd., 80 Strand, London WC2R 0RL, England
Penguin Group Ireland, 25 St. Stephen's Green, Dublin 2, Ireland (a division of Penguin Books Ltd.)
Penguin Group (Australia), 250 Camberwell Road, Camberwell, Victoria 3124, Australia
(a division of Pearson Australia Group Pty. Ltd.)
Penguin Books India Pvt. Ltd., 11 Community Centre, Panchsheel Park, New Delhi—110 017, India
Penguin Group (NZ), 67 Apollo Drive, Rosedale, Auckland 0632, New Zealand
(a division of Pearson New Zealand Ltd.)
Penguin Books (South Africa) (Pty.) Ltd., 24 Sturdee Avenue, Rosebank, Johannesburg 2196,
South Africa

Penguin Books Ltd., Registered Offices: 80 Strand, London WC2R 0RL, England

This book is an original publication of The Berkley Publishing Group.

PUBLISHER's NOTE: Every effort has been made to ensure that the information contained in this book is complete and accurate. However, neither the publisher nor the authors are engaged in rendering professional advice or services to the individual reader. The ideas, procedures, and suggestions contained in this book are not intended as a substitute for consulting with your physician. All matters regarding your health require medical supervision. Neither the authors nor the publisher shall be liable or responsible for any loss or damage allegedly arising from any information or suggestion in this book.

The recipes contained in this book are to be followed exactly as written. The publisher is not responsible for your specific health or allergy needs that may require medical supervision. The publisher is not responsible for any adverse reactions to the recipes contained in this book.

The publisher does not have any control over and does not assume responsibility for author or third-party websites or their content.

PRINTING HISTORY
Berkley trade paperback edition / January 2012

Library of Congress Cataloging-in-Publication Data

Anderson, James W.
  The simple diet : a doctor's science-based plan / James W. Anderson and Nancy J. Gustafson.
    p. cm.
  ISBN 978-0-425-24106-6 (pbk.)
  1. Weight loss—Popular works. 2. Reducing diets—Popular works. 3. Nutrition—Popular
works. 4. Exercise—Popular works. I. Gustafson, Nancy J. II. Title.
  RM222.2.A515 2012
  613.7'12—dc23
                        2011032310

PRINTED IN THE UNITED STATES OF AMERICA

10  9  8  7  6  5  4  3  2  1

*I dedicate this book to my loving family: Gay, Kathy, Steve, Tom, Anne, Allison, Emily, Caroline, Camille, and Brielle, who continue to inspire me. I also am deeply indebted to my many patients who have encouraged and worked with me as I have asked them to make big changes in their lifestyle.*

—James W. Anderson

*To my wonderful husband, children, and children-in-law; for their love, support, and patience.*

—Nancy J. Gustafson

# Acknowledgments

I (James W. Anderson) appreciate the encouragement of Bill Gottlieb and the assistance of Allison Kroll and Lacey Lamb.

The success stories that you read about in this book were all patients I worked with directly. While there are many diet programs and meal replacements available, a number of these participants achieved their results using Health Management Resources (HMR) meal replacements while following the HMR Program. Although the individual stories are based on patients I have treated, the names, ages, occupations, and other details have been modified to protect the identity of these individuals.

We appreciate the diligent and insightful editing of Denise Silvestro, Meredith Giordan, Kate Ritchey, and Jessica McDonnell. The support, editorial help, and encouragement of our agent, Stephany Evans, was invaluable.

# Contents

# Contents

# Meet Your Future

If losing weight were easy, we'd all look fabulous and I would have spent most of my research life trying to solve another problem. But losing weight *is* difficult—in fact, for many people, it's almost impossible—which is why I've spent most of my career studying how to effectively reverse overweight and the diseases it causes or complicates. I've been particularly interested in reversing obesity, defined as carrying 30 or more extra pounds.

Medically, obesity puts you at higher risk for heart attack, stroke, high blood pressure, diabetes, cancer, and other life-threatening health conditions. Socially, it stops you from easily participating in everyday activities, whether it's romping with your kids or grandkids or fitting comfortably into an airplane seat on your next vacation. Emotionally, it sabotages your self-image. And that includes feeling like a failure every time you blow a diet, which, if you're like most obese people, is over and over again. Failure feels awful. Why even bother starting another diet?

This book tells you that weight-loss failure does not have to be your destiny. I'll tell you about a science-based method for weight-loss success for anyone who needs to lose moderate to large amounts of weight. Yes, losing a lot of weight takes dedication, courage, and effort, but it *can* be done if you follow the right program.

# Diabesity— From the Lab to the Clinic

Obesity and diabetes are like conjoined twins—they are almost inseparable. In medical school, I developed a commitment to searching for a cure for diabetes. My first efforts were in the biochemistry laboratory at Northwestern University, then at Mayo Clinic, at the U.S. Army Nutrition Laboratory, at the University of California, San Francisco, and, for the last thirty-eight years, at the University of Kentucky.

In the lab, I explored mechanisms contributing to diabetes, obesity, and blood lipid problems. As I began treating patients with diabetes in the clinic, I quickly learned that 80 percent were obese. This led me to address the obesity issue. As we brought the research ward experience to the clinic, we developed very-low-calorie diets using meal replacements. For my first fifteen years in Kentucky, I treated obese diabetic individuals in the research ward and in the VA Diabetes Clinic with very-low-calorie (under 800 calorie) and low-calorie (800–1,200 calorie) diets, and found that effective weight loss could produce a "cure" for some obese diabetic individuals.

In 1985, I engineered the partnership between Health Management Resources (HMR) and the University of Kentucky. Over the next twenty-five years, as medical director of the HMR Program for Weight Management at the University of Kentucky (hereafter called "the program"), I worked closely with individuals enrolled in the program, and many of the scientific articles I have published have been related to my experiences with these individuals. Similarly, while all of the case studies presented in this book are composites, they are based on real people I have worked with, and many of them used meal replacement products from the program to achieve their weight loss. My work with the program validated and extended what I had learned from working with obese individuals throughout my career. This book is an outgrowth of these many years of experience in this field of study. This includes over ten thousand obese patients treated at the university or VA clinic and hospital and over five thousand patients treated in the program.

In addition to my academic and professional experiences, I also knew about obesity personally. When I was growing up, my dad stood out in a crowd, not because of his five foot three height, but because of his 235-pound weight; he was severely obese. My mother also was chunky. With my eighty-hour work weeks and extensive national and international travel, I also accumulated weight, and for a short period was on the cusp of obesity at 193 pounds, which is too much for my frame. This heightened my focus on obesity. I dropped down to 155 pounds when I started the program in 1985, but to be frank, I have carried 173 to 187 pounds for most of my adult life. I will also share with you many practical tips and how I dropped 30 pounds while writing this book.

Like my dad, I love to eat, and like my mom, I love to cook. In the early 1980s, I was also researching the health benefits of low-fat, high-fiber diets in addition to my obesity research. As I began developing these diets, I began developing recipes. I became known as Dr. Oat Bran because I helped popularize oat bran. My first oat-bran muffins were like hockey pucks, but I eventually learned how to make tasty muffins that people still eat and brag about because of the effects on their blood cholesterol levels. I have published several hundred recipes and have included a number of shake and entrée recipes in this book for you to enjoy.

The Simple Diet is an outgrowth of my research related to obesity, diabetes, high blood fats, and pursuit of the optimal diet for everyone. The goals of this book are to make it easy for you to lose weight safely and effectively, and to develop a lifestyle change in order to manage your weight long-term. I hope to empower you to lose your excess weight and keep it off.

*Jan, a charismatic fifty-year-old college dean from Georgia, weighed in at 316 pounds, with a height of five feet seven inches. She had a large frame, and a health-promoting weight for her would be about 160 pounds. At her initial evaluation, she had high blood pressure, arthritis, high blood cholesterol, and varicose veins.*

*This charming, talkative woman with blue-gray eyes and blond hair had taken a leave of absence for one academic year and was in Kentucky to be with and care for her mother, who had terminal cancer. When she heard about the program, she recognized an opportunity to do something for herself as well. She jumped into the*

*program with both feet and followed it religiously, using
meal replacements, fruits, and vegetables while gradually
increasing her physical activity.*

*Jan flagged me down in the hall about five months after I
had done her initial exam. I didn't recognize her, and she
quickly let me know that she had lost 110 pounds and was at
her lowest weight since before her last pregnancy. She had
stopped all her medicines—for blood pressure, high
cholesterol, and arthritis. She now walked three miles daily
and worked out at the gym three times a week. She looked
firm and fit. Because her mother had recently died, she was
returning to her college, where her faculty and staff had not
seen her since she began the program. Only a secretary and
one other person knew what she was doing. They were
planning to do a video of her return to school! At 206
pounds, she was a striking woman with a winning smile and
an engaging personality. And she assured me that she was
sticking with the program and was determined to reach her
goal weight before the new school year started.*

## The Best Weight-Loss Value

A quick look at the statistics tells us that traditional diets don't
produce the results most obese people need. In a study recently
published in a premier medical journal, the *Journal of the American Medical Association*, the average overweight person following
one of three popular diets with nutrition counseling lost an average of 7.2 pounds in six months and regained almost a pound at
the end of the year.[1] That's not very encouraging!

People who follow the Simple Diet fare much better. Of the hundred-plus articles I've published about obesity, 25 percent of them have related to this type of weight-loss program, so the results are well documented. The average person who participates in the program using a combination of meal replacements, fruits, and vegetables for a minimum of nine weeks loses 42 pounds.[2]

Our most recent studies have focused on a group of people we call the 100-Pound Club—two hundred and fifty people who have lost 100 pounds or more on the program. All of these people were severely obese and needed to lose at least 100 pounds to preserve their health. Again, with a program that used varying combinations of meal replacements, fruits, and vegetables, people in the 100-Pound Club lost an average of 50 pounds in just twelve weeks, and lost an average of 100 pounds in twenty-four weeks. Some went on to lose another 50 to 200 pounds or more.[3] We are seeing more and more people who are losing large amounts of weight using the Simple Diet approach. Now you can do this, too.

But not everyone needs to lose 100 pounds. Hundreds of people are members of the 50-Pound Club, having lost 50 pounds or more using the same approach. Would you like to join one of these clubs? Do you have 30, 50, 100, or more pounds you'd like to lose—and keep off? You've come to the right place. If you're ready to start the program, then:

- you won't need dangerous (and expensive) weight-loss surgery;
- you won't need to take (expensive) weight-loss drugs and suffer from their unpleasant or hazardous side effects; and

- you won't need to check in to an (expensive) weight-loss spa.

And don't worry—club members don't have to be paragons of virtue and willpower. They all feel the same way you do about eating practically nothing but rice cakes and celery, or following a diet with too many rules. Diets that are complicated or rely on deprivation don't work, at least not for long.

The Simple Diet is easy to follow. It is based on meal replacements—eating preportioned entrées, shakes, and other packaged foods—and fruits and vegetables. But instead of making you join a program that restricts you to its special foods, we will tell you all you need to know to be able to pick from more than two hundred appropriate meal replacements, and give you a whole selection of choices that are available in grocery and convenience stores across the country.

Instead of trying to figure out which foods are "good" or "bad," which are "allowed" or "forbidden," you simply enjoy nutritionally balanced, delicious, premeasured meal replacements along with your favorite fruits and vegetables. And you'll be amazed as pounds fall off easily, at an average of two to three pounds per week, week after week. We'll also share with you how you can talk to yourself (self-talk) in a manner that helps you keep a positive can-do attitude. Each chapter includes "I can do . . ." statements to help you get started on your self-talk.

The First Phase of the Simple Diet is the intensive weight-loss phase, where you are using meal replacements, fruits, and vegetables; increasing your physical activity; and learning the skills of health and weight management. As you get closer to your goal weight, you transition to the Second Phase, the health and weight management phase. In the Second Phase, you continue your physical activity and lifestyle skills while using fewer meal replacements, still enjoying fruits and vegetables, and gradually introducing a greater variety of low-fat, high-fiber foods. We'll give you a Green Light Calorie Guide to help you select foods that are low in calories, fats, and sugars and high in fiber. Near the end of the book, we'll ask you to think beyond weight to lifetime health habits, and we'll tell you about the Simple Lifetime Diet—a diet that returns you to a fully balanced, health-promoting diet for life (and one your family can begin immediately).

The Simple Diet includes regular physical activity to achieve and maintain a good to excellent level of fitness and health. You'll need to increase your physical activity to walking about two miles per day, or the equivalent in other forms of physical activity. Of course you will do this gradually; if you currently consider yourself to be somewhat of a couch potato, you will start with baby steps. You also will weigh yourself regularly and will discover that the scale is your friend (or at least a useful tool), not your enemy. And I'll show you the importance of keeping records. Just like using your golf or bowling scores to better your game, keeping weight and health records helps you assess how you are doing with the diet and see if changes are needed.

## Health and Weight Management

We often hear that people who lose a lot of weight regain most of it within a few years. The research shows that this dismal— and frankly dispiriting—outcome is not inevitable. We have recently analyzed data from 180 individuals who lost an average of 65 pounds at different weight-loss clinics around the country that use a weight-loss approach similar to the Simple Diet. After five years, about 20 percent of the individuals regained all their weight, but 25 percent of participants maintained average weight losses of 56 pounds at five years, and *most* of the participants were maintaining *more than half* of their weight loss after five years.[4] Similarly, the 118 charter members of the 100-Pound Club lost 134 pounds and are keeping off 65 pounds after five years.[5]

The secret to success for many of the 100-Pound Club members is the continued use of meal replacements and generous consumption of fruits and vegetables over the years. Use of shakes or preportioned entrées is a valuable weight management tool for ongoing use or for regrouping after a holiday or special event when a few pounds creep back. I personally have used meal replacements on an almost daily basis for more than twenty-five years.

Why are meal replacements so effective? Hundreds of studies in the field of behavioral science show that it's very difficult to stop a bad habit—whether it's smoking, chewing your nails, or overeating—by just deciding to stop. One decision cannot reverse years (or decades) of learned behaviors and habits. What behavioral scientists have discovered, however, is that it's easier to *exchange* one behavior for another. By following the Simple Diet, you will be exchanging calorie-laden meals for meal replacements. You'll also learn how to stay active to burn calories, keep everyday health records for instant feedback on progress or setbacks, and build social support.

The Simple Diet has worked for thousands of obese and extremely obese people, and it can and will work for you—safely, effectively, economically. Many people have changed their lives by using this program. They're thinner, healthier, and happier. Now it's your turn!

## "I can use the Simple Diet to become healthier and feel better."

# Obesity and Extreme Obesity: A Big Problem

This book is not just for people looking to lose five pounds for their class reunion or their daughter's wedding. It's not just for people who want to tone their trouble spots or fit into their skinny jeans. Even though these people may benefit from this book, too, *The Simple Diet* is really for the millions of Americans who are 30 or more pounds above a health-promoting weight and are ready to do something about it.

We may not like the word, but if you are 30 pounds overweight, you are clinically obese, and 90 pounds overweight puts you in the extreme obesity category. Both conditions put you at a higher risk for a host of medical problems. Severe obesity has increased sixfold in the United States in the last fifty years. Obesity is *the* major health problem in the United States and *the* leading cause of preventable death. Obesity is the major cause of diabetes, and is responsible for one-third of all heart attacks. About 40 percent of American schoolchildren are overweight or obese, and 65 percent of adults are overweight or obese.

Could we have imagined, even twenty years ago, popular television programs featuring extremely obese individuals competing to lose the most weight, or a British chef attempting to school American children on healthy eating habits? These are signs of our times. At the present rate of gain, unless dramatic public health interventions occur (imagine that!), an estimated 86 percent of Americans will be overweight or obese by 2030.[6]

Although about 40 percent of Americans are currently on a weight-loss diet, the results are not evident. Clearly, we need a better strategy to help people better manage their weight.

## Obesity and Your Health

Obesity is a major cause of health problems. You probably know a lot of women who have gained 15 pounds since high school, but you may not know that even this small weight gain doubles their risk for developing diabetes. For guys, a 35-pound weight gain after high school triples their risk for getting diabetes. Overall, obesity is directly related to 80 percent of diabetes, and losing the extra pounds consistently reverses the disease.

The higher the adult weight, the higher the risk for developing diabetes. Severely obese individuals are seventeen times more likely to develop diabetes than very slender people. People who gain substantial weight after high school and are severely obese are *ninety times* more likely to develop diabetes than slender individuals.[7] In addition, overweight or obesity contributes to 14 percent of all cancer deaths in men and to 20 percent in women.[8]

In the United States, more women die from heart disease than men. While coronary heart disease is decreasing in men, it continues to increase in women. Obesity is a major contributor to heart attacks in women. The pioneering studies of JoAnn Manson, MD, of Harvard University document that very slender women have the lowest risk for heart attacks. These studies also show that overweight women are at greater than threefold risk, and mildly obese women have a sixfold risk. In other words, a woman who is more than 30 pounds overweight is six times more likely to have a heart attack than a slender woman.[9]

Obese individuals also suffer more from high blood pressure, strokes, high blood cholesterol, cancer, arthritis, breathing problems, indigestion, varicose veins, immune disorders (like lupus), infections (like recurrent sinus problems), and a lot of other medical problems. They also experience decreased energy, depression, and low self-esteem. Their hospital stays are riskier. Their health care costs are higher. And their lives are shorter. Below is just a partial list of health problems associated with overweight and obesity.

- Diabetes
- Heart disease
- Hypertension
- Sleep apnea
- Degenerative joint disease
- Gallbladder disease
- Dyslipidemia
- Infertility
- Depression
- Psychosocial pain
- Premature death
- Gastroesophageal reflux disease
- Nonalcoholic fatty liver disease
- Lower cognitive performance
- Certain forms of cancer (especially breast cancer)
- Gout
- Chronic low-grade inflammation
- Reduced immune responsiveness
- More complications with pregnancy
- Varicose vein disease

For women of childbearing age, obesity reduces fertility and increases risk of pregnancy complications. Pregnant women who are severely obese are eight times more likely to develop gestational diabetes (high blood sugar during pregnancy). Pregnant women who are moderately obese are three times as likely to develop preeclampsia, a condition that can be fatal for mother and baby if left untreated. Obese women also have cesarean section deliveries more frequently than non-obese women.

Until recently, extreme obesity (also called severe or morbid obesity) was considered to be a rare condition. But rates are skyrocketing, with the number of extremely obese Americans six times higher than they were in the 1960s. What's going on?

## Genes or Jeans?

My mom was chunky and my dad was severely obese—I don't stand a chance of being skinny, right? Not so! All of us inherit some bad genes and some good genes. But we need to play the hand we are dealt.

Based on all I've studied, I believe genes account for about 40 percent of the risk for obesity. Our genes haven't changed much in the ten thousand years since our ancestors were hunter-gatherers scrounging for food and scurrying away from predators to avoid becoming *their* food. The explosive worldwide increase in obesity in the last few decades does not relate to changes in our genes; it relates to changes in our *environment*.

By environment, I don't mean global warming. I mean the social and cultural environment—where we live and how we live. *Where* we live, there's more food than ever before: supersized, calorie-laden food readily available at the gas station, the fast-food restaurant, the supermarket, the mini-mart, the food court in the mall, the office break room, and in most homes. (Recently I was in a furniture store that regularly serves pastries and coffee to shoppers.) *How* we live is by moving less and burning fewer calories, from changing channels with the remote control to lowering the car window by pushing a button. Genes load the gun, but environment pulls the trigger.

Many factors contribute to obesity. Clearly, high fat and sugar intake coupled with a low fiber intake are positively related to weight gain; high intakes of whole grains, fruits, and vegetables protect us from obesity. Our general inactivity is also a major factor. Perhaps a typical Nebraska farmer walked a hundred miles a week in 1900, but many folks don't walk a hundred miles in six months or even a year now. Many in our social circles, our family members and friends, are overweight and provide constant encouragement and permission for us to overeat. Poor stress management, inadequate sleep, and lack of time for meditation and reflection also contribute. Other factors that may contribute to weight gain are medications (such as antidepressants and antihistamines), physical limitations, abuse as a child, and illness. So weight management presents a challenge for virtually all Americans.

## Now—The Simple Diet

Although I could go on about the health risks of obesity, let me emphasize the good news: Following the Simple Diet can lessen and even reverse these conditions. With the Simple Diet, thousands of people have lowered their blood pressure and blood cholesterol levels, their diabetes has disappeared, and they are able to feel better about themselves and enjoy life more. I understand that many extremely obese people don't trust that they have the willpower to lose weight. They believe that even if they try, they're going to fail. But I've spent my medical career helping people lose weight and have seen all the positive results. It all begins with reading and putting into practice the scientifically proven advice in this book. Robbie's and Emily's stories illustrate the kind of success I'm talking about.

*Robbie, a forty-nine-year-old high school science teacher, came to see me with a host of medical problems in addition to his severe obesity. At his evaluation, he was six feet tall and 340 pounds. He had diabetes, hypertension, lipid abnormalities, fatty liver disease, and sleep apnea. He used a CPAP machine every night for his sleep apnea and was taking eight prescription medications, which cost him $700 each month. He was a gregarious, outgoing person who was full of life.*

*Robbie started the program using three shakes plus two entrées daily and did extremely well. He lost 120 pounds in twenty-seven weeks, and we discontinued all his medications and the CPAP machine during this period. His diabetes went into remission, with normal blood glucose values on no medication. His hypertension disappeared (his final blood pressure on no medication was 100/64), and all his blood lipids and liver function tests were normal. He had another sleep test in the sleep laboratory and he had no evidence of sleep apnea.*

*Over this period, I saw Robbie on about twenty occasions, and at each visit he expressed profound gratitude for the program. He gave testimonials at his church about his weight loss.* The Saturday Evening Post *wanted to do a story about him, so he came in for photographs and brought his pre-weight-loss pants. Just like the famous weight-loss advertisements I'm sure you've seen, he was able to fit his entire person into one leg of his old pants.*

*At eighteen months after leaving the weight-loss program, he is at 224 pounds and doing very well. He continues to walk three miles per day and uses two shakes and one entrée each day. He consumes about ten servings of fruits and vegetables per day, and his diabetes is well controlled on one medication (metformin) that acts to prevent his more severe diabetes from coming back.*

*Emily came in to see me before Christmas. This twenty-seven-year-old CPA had just gotten engaged to another accountant and was planning to be married the next June. At five feet five inches tall, she weighed 197 pounds. She wanted to lose 50 pounds before her wedding, and we decided this was a reasonable goal.*

*Emily was a serious-minded person, quiet and shy. She had become chubby in college, and had compensated, in part, by being the best student in her class. She had sailed through college in three years, aced her CPA exam, and landed a job in a top accounting firm, where she met Arnold. Now they wanted to get married and raise little "bean counters."*

*She started the program on January 5, using three shakes and two entrées daily. She also spent an hour at the gym six days a week. Like many accountants, she was a good record keeper and brought in Excel spreadsheets of her meal replacement use and physical activity each week.*

*Emily lost 50 pounds in seventeen weeks. She reported "perfect scores" for using five meal replacements daily with no other food, and exceeded the recommended physical activity of walking fourteen miles per week (her average was twenty-eight miles per week). In May, she transitioned to the Second Phase for health and weight management and lost another eight pounds before her wedding. She was a trim and fit bride at 139 pounds—her lowest weight since eighth grade.*

You, too, can enjoy the weight-loss success that Robbie and Emily experienced. Both of these people had positive can-do attitudes. In this book, I will outline the Simple Diet's Six Keys to Intensive Weight Loss. Following these simple prescriptions will put you on your way to fast, significant, and lasting weight loss. The Simple Diet is as easy as 1, 2, 3.

## "I can eat two nutritious entrées, drink three tasty shakes, and consume five servings of healthful fruits and vegetables daily."

# Discovering
# the Solution:
# The Simple Diet

Y

ou and I have been on diets before. Many of us have even lost 30, 40, or 50 pounds. But it was a major struggle, right? Then, didn't the lost weight come back? Sometimes we even gained *additional* weight. Well, now there's a better strategy for losing weight and keeping it off. We'll get to the details later, but let me show you some of the scientific evidence to support this claim.

I believe the Simple Diet is the most effective nonsurgical weight-loss and weight management approach that has ever been reported. These results have been achieved with minimal side effects and without drugs or surgery.

The figure on the next page compares the average weight losses for obese people participating in various programs that promote a healthy diet and lifestyle. To clarify, the average participant entering these programs weighed about 200 pounds and was 60 pounds above a non-obese weight. Over six months, the average participant lost between 2 and 34 pounds with these interventions: dietitian counseling,[10] Slim-Fast,[11] Weight Watchers,[12] Jenny Craig,[13] Medifast,[14] and the Simple Diet.[15]

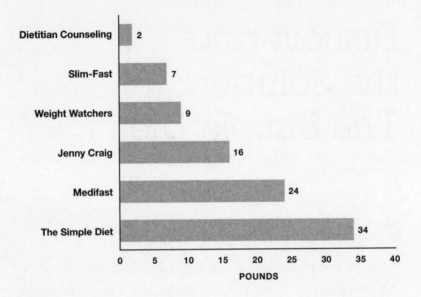

What accounts for such large differences in weight loss from program to program? Research shows that people lose substantially more weight when they follow a highly structured program using meal replacements. Counseling about healthy eating is not nearly as effective as removing any guesswork about appropriate foods or portions by instituting or encouraging the use of meal replacements.

The Simple Diet is clearly more effective than other programs using meal replacements because of its unique approach and because of the accountability that is strongly encouraged and supported by the use of food records. Successful individuals in the program use a minimum of five meal replacements and five servings of fruits and vegetables and walk two miles daily to achieve their weight goals. Given an array of foods to choose from, most people on the program find it easy to stay on the Simple Diet and can avoid foods not on the diet. Now you can benefit from this program, too.

I've devoted my entire medical career to treating people with diabetes and other health problems caused by obesity and looking for new and better ways to help them lose weight and regain health. I *know* the Simple Diet works because I've helped over 250 patients lose 100 pounds or more and keep most of it off. In addition, I've helped close to fifteen thousand others shed lesser but still large amounts of weight. I'd like to share some of that story with you here.

# The Devastation of Diabetes

In 1959, as a junior medical student attending Northwestern University Medical School in Chicago, Illinois, I was assigned to the diabetes service at Passavant Memorial Hospital. I helped care for all the patients with diabetes in the hospital and supervised their diabetes management.

Diabetes is a disease of high blood sugar levels. In type 1 diabetes (an autoimmune disease that usually afflicts the young), the pancreas doesn't make enough insulin, a hormone that directs sugar into the cells. In type 2 diabetes (a lifestyle disease that used to mostly afflict the middle-aged and elderly, but now is increasingly common among children, teenagers, and young adults), the cells in muscles and other parts of the body become resistant to insulin, so that the insulin-generating pancreas has to make more and more insulin and eventually wears out.

Over time, high blood sugar levels in people with diabetes damage blood vessels. This results in heart attacks or strokes; kidney problems; blindness; nerve damage with burning, tingling, or numbness; and even amputation of disease-ravaged feet. My patients at Passavant Memorial Hospital suffered from all these conditions and more.

I soon realized that I wanted to do whatever I could to help patients avoid these types of problems. That meant teaching them to manage their diabetes effectively, with medications and with diet.

Even in 1959, studies had shown that patients could manage diabetes effectively with dietary changes. And type 2 diabetes was mostly a disease of people who were overweight or obese, suggesting that it could be delayed or avoided altogether by correcting obesity. *Could* type 2 diabetes be stopped or reversed if people lost weight? I was determined to answer that question.

## Fasting and Weight Loss

I earned my MD degree from Northwestern University and completed my medical training in endocrinology as a fellow at the Mayo Clinic in Rochester, Minnesota. All the while, my research focused on the effects of dietary change and weight loss on diabetes and other weight-related conditions.

During the Vietnam War, I joined the Army and was stationed at the Fitzsimons Army Medical Center in Denver, Colorado. My medical colleagues and I were assigned to the Army Nutrition Laboratory. (This facility was called the Nut Lab, a nickname that has afflicted me ever since; my blog address is NutDoc.)

Our assignment: to develop an ideal meal replacement (Meal, Ready-to-Eat, or MRE) for soldiers in the field. The meal replacement needed to be lightweight, easy to prepare, and nutritionally complete so that soldiers could eat it, unsupplemented, if circumstances demanded, over many weeks or months without detrimental effects. My role was to learn how calorie restriction—whether on the battlefield or in everyday life—leads people to lose weight, and what happens to them as they do. And so began my research into fasting for weight loss.

In those days, total fasting—eating no food whatsoever—was becoming a popular method for losing large amounts of weight. But my colleagues and I knew total fasting might be dangerous, so we kept close tabs on our fasting patients in the research unit of the Army Nutrition Laboratory, monitoring blood pressure, blood chemistry, and any other physical changes.

I specifically remember one patient, an Army sergeant who was not assigned overseas duty because he was obese. The Army put him in the hospital for a total fast. The sergeant lost weight quickly, was discharged from the hospital, and went right back to gaining weight. That's when he ended up in our unit.

I talked with the sergeant about his eating habits, wondering how he could gain so much weight in such a short period of time. I asked him to describe a typical breakfast. "Well, let's see, doc," he said. "For breakfast, I usually have a dozen eggs, a pound of bacon, and a loaf of toast."

Fasting may have been effective over a short term. But we learned that unless eating *habits* change, there was no long-term weight loss. We also learned that total fasting is unsafe for several reasons (a discovery that would later help my colleagues and me design safer, more effective diets and meal replacements for weight loss).

During total fasting, the body loses the mineral potassium at a rapid rate, leading to fainting, heart irregularities, weakness, and fatigue. Total fasting also causes the body to devour muscle tissue for protein, including heart tissue. Combined with potassium deficiency, this effect can lead to heart irregularities and even death. Surprisingly, total fasting also caused patients to become resistant to insulin, a condition that precedes the development of diabetes. (In contrast, when we fed patients a very-low-calorie diet of 500 calories daily that included some carbohydrate, they remained sensitive to insulin.)

Total fasting was clearly not a healthy solution for weight loss. In fact, it created even more problems for patients.

## Very-Low-Calorie Diets

My two years of research on fasting and meal replacements in the Army would stimulate and direct my research interests for the next forty years.

After seeing the positive effects of very-low-calorie diets (VLCDs) compared with total fasting in our Army studies, I pursued this line of research when I was discharged, first at the University of California Medical School in San Francisco, and then at the University of Kentucky College of Medicine in Lexington, where much of both my clinical work with patients and formal research has taken place since 1973.

VLCDs provide fewer than 800 calories daily, from either whole food or meal replacements. In the late 1970s and early 1980s, we tested VLCDs made up of carefully selected foods in the hospital setting. The most successful food-based VLCD during this time provided adequate potassium to stave off the effects of potassium loss and ample carbohydrate and protein for energy and muscle maintenance.

During this same period, we also discovered that including generous amounts of dietary fiber in the VLCD reduced hunger and increased satiety levels (satisfaction after a meal) for our patients trying to lose weight. Dietary fiber is the indigestible portion of plant foods; fruits, vegetables, and whole grains are high in dietary fiber.

In one of the studies of weight-loss approaches for obese men with diabetes, we compared the safety and weight-loss effectiveness of high-carbohydrate, high-fiber diets at four different calorie levels. This study included both an 800-calorie diet group and a 500- to 600-VLCD group. Predictably, patients in the lower calorie ranges lost the most weight. But—a very interesting finding—weight losses on the 800-calorie and the VLCD were similar: an average of 6.4 pounds per week for patients on the 800-calorie diet and 6.5 pounds per week for patients on the VLCD. For both groups, average insulin doses dropped 60 percent and need for oral diabetes medication decreased about 70 percent. The blood glucose value declined 30 percent despite the large reduction in insulin and oral diabetes medication. Blood cholesterol levels and levels of other dangerous blood fats also fell on both diets.[16]

*Johnny was one of the men assigned to the 800-calorie diet in this study. He was a successful hog farmer from Arkansas who in 1981 came to our VA hospital in Kentucky because he heard we were helping people with diabetes lose weight and stop taking insulin. Johnny had been an outstanding football player in high school and college, but he had never changed his eating habits when he stopped playing football.*

*At age forty-nine and six feet two inches tall, Johnny weighed 340 pounds. He had developed type 2 diabetes at the age of thirty-four. When I first saw him, he had been taking insulin for four years, using ninety units of insulin before each meal—a dose four times the typical dose for someone his size.*

*Johnny checked into the hospital well after dinner, because he had wanted his "last meal" (and a few beers, too) before surrendering to the study. He would start the 800-calorie diet in the morning.*

*Usually, I reduced insulin doses by about 50 percent when my patients started this type of diet, then adjusted downward as needed. However, I suspected Johnny enjoyed "eating up" to his ninety units of insulin and probably didn't need insulin at all, so I stopped his insulin cold turkey.*

*We watched Johnny closely the next day, checking his blood sugar levels several times. On the second morning, thirty-six hours after checking in to the hospital, his fasting blood sugar level was in the normal range. Over the next two weeks, while losing 1.3 pounds per day, or 9 pounds per week, all his blood sugar values were in the normal range. He was incredulous that he did not have to take insulin. His blood pressure dropped into the normal range, and we reduced his blood pressure medicine from four tablets a day to one. His blood levels of triglycerides—a heart-threatening fat—decreased from 627 mg/dl on the first morning to normal values of 139 mg/dl before he left the hospital.*

*Johnny went home on one diabetes tablet and one blood pressure pill per day.*

# The Emergence of Meal Replacements

In the 1980s, we started experimenting with using meal replacements in the form of liquid shakes for patients on the VLCD. My colleagues and I at the University of Kentucky carefully recorded results with different formulas and modified the types of meal replacements we used.

When we talk about meal replacements, we are including anything from powdered or liquid shakes to prepackaged entrées (similar to frozen dinners). Properly designed, meal replacements have the advantage of being formulated to provide the right amount of protein, carbohydrate, potassium, and other nutrients—all at a low-calorie level—allowing rapid but safe weight loss. A huge benefit of quality meal replacements is that they are a known quantity; they can eliminate any potential error in choice of foods and maximize nutritional intake for the limited number of calories consumed. By using meal replacements, we were able to offer VLCDs outside of the hospital setting.

I wasn't the only researcher studying VLCDs in the 1980s. Other teams of scientists were noticing that their weight-loss patients lost weight rapidly and experienced fewer side effects when they used VLCDs instead of total fasting. Soon the findings from the scientific community trickled down to dieters— and VLCD liquid diets swept the country and the world.

Containing 330 calories daily, the Cambridge Diet was all the rage in Europe. OPTIFAST launched a 420-calorie diet that was later made infamous when Oprah Winfrey announced a 67-pound weight loss on television—and then regained all of the weight.

Unfortunately, some of the meal replacements on the market were nutritionally inadequate and caused serious side effects and even deaths. Others were distributed without adequate supervision of the person losing weight. Or they lacked the context of a comprehensive approach that included exercise, social support, and a transition to weight maintenance.

In 1985, my colleagues and I at the University of Kentucky joined forces with Health Management Resources (HMR). We began offering a comprehensive, shake-based VLCD program on an outpatient basis for all the obese individuals we were treating, whether they had diabetes or not. The VLCD was carefully formulated, providing 520 calories daily, adequate potassium, high-quality protein, and as much carbohydrate as the calorie level would allow. I saw patients once weekly in the clinic, and we checked their blood chemistries every other week. We encouraged patients to be physically active, to keep an ongoing record of their use of meal replacements and their other food intake, and to attend weekly classes for encouragement and support.

Our program was increasingly successful. My patients were losing weight and reducing their medications. Our first report of the program's success appeared in the *Journal of the American Dietetic Association* in 1991, where we reported results for the first hundred patients who enrolled in the program. Women in the program lost an average of 42 pounds in seventeen weeks; men lost an average of 41 pounds in twelve weeks. Both average blood cholesterol and blood sugar levels dropped significantly.[17]

In another study, published in the *American Journal of Clinical Nutrition* the following year, eighty extremely obese patients had similar results: They lost an average of 78 pounds in twenty-six weeks and reduced their blood pressure, blood sugar, and cholesterol levels.[18]

These and other published studies all showed our patients were making huge strides in weight loss and improved health.

# From Very-Low-Calorie to Low-Calorie Diets

While we were offering VLCDs for our patients, we also did research with low-calorie diets, which provide 800 to 1,200 calories daily. We were very pleased with the results achieved by our patients with diabetes who participated in our early research work using these diets. During their weight-loss phase, their average fasting blood glucose values dropped 28 percent, and the hemoglobin A1C (a measure of average blood glucose over the last two to three months) decreased 21 percent. These improvements in blood glucose levels occurred while decreasing average insulin doses by 60 percent and oral diabetes medicines by 71 percent.[19] By 1992, we were recommending low-calorie diets rather than VLCDs for virtually all of our patients.

From our earlier studies, we had seen that patients on a food-based 800-calorie diet lost just as much weight as patients on a VLCD. My experiences treating a mother-daughter duo showed me that adding more calories could still support large weight losses. While Helen lost weight on a VLCD, her daughter, Pam, lost 180 pounds in sixty-two weeks on a low-calorie diet.

*Helen was a forty-four-year-old elementary education teacher whose father had been a volunteer in our weight-loss studies with diabetic individuals conducted on the research ward at the VA hospital. Her daughter, Pam, thirteen years old, was her only child. The two of them had been very close since Helen's husband had left the family ten years earlier.*

*Helen wanted to lose 100 pounds, and she wanted us to help Pam, who, at five feet three inches, weighed 340 pounds. We had never treated a thirteen-year-old with a VLCD, so we decided to treat her with a more liberal 800 calories and 80 grams of protein daily and monitored her closely.*

*Helen was a no-nonsense person who reminded me of drill sergeants I had known in the military. She was stocky, with short brown hair. Her attire was more functional than stylish. At her initial visit, she weighed 250 pounds at five feet four inches tall. She had high blood pressure, high blood triglyceride levels, and osteoarthritis.*

*Pam was a shy, introverted teenager. She was teased at school about her weight, and over time voiced resentment and anger about this. She did not pay much attention to what she wore, and her brown hair looked like she'd cut it herself— without a mirror.*

*Helen and Pam attended weight-loss classes together, kept complete records, and rarely missed a session. They started walking together after school, and as Pam became more mobile, they would walk three miles in ninety minutes, with their time dropping to fifty-five minutes as they lost weight. They both followed the diet religiously.*

*Helen lost 90 pounds in twenty-eight weeks. We stopped*

*her blood pressure medication. Her triglycerides decreased from 270 mg/dl to 110 mg/dl. And her demeanor in class changed—from a serious-minded, sober person who didn't have much to smile about to an enthusiastic and fun person. After about two months, she insisted on giving me a bear hug every time she saw me.*

*Pam lost 180 pounds over sixty-two weeks—more than half her initial body weight. We monitored her for any adverse symptoms, but observed no problems. After her mother reached her goal weight, she continued to go to class with her daughter to provide support. However, Pam was her own person and developed her independence during this time period. She became more talkative in class and was well liked by her weight-loss classmates.*

*Both Helen and Pam remained in the program for one more year after Pam achieved her maximum weight loss. I saw Helen about ten years later—she was doing well and appeared to be keeping much of her weight off. I saw Pam fourteen years later, at age twenty-eight. We did not have time to talk very long, but she indicated that she was happily married. She appeared to weigh about 200 pounds.*

*I saw Pam again four years after that, at age thirty-two— eighteen years after she and her mother had completed the program. She came up, gave me one of her mother's bear hugs, and said, "Dr. Anderson, you saved my life." At the time she was four months pregnant with her second child. She reported that her pre-pregnancy weight was about 200 pounds, at five feet five inches tall.*

[
CAUTION: While we have used this diet effectively for hundreds of teenagers in our clinic under close medical supervision, teenagers should not embark on the Simple Diet without careful monitoring by an experienced physician.
]

The particulars of Pam's weight-loss story stuck with me. She lost more weight overall than her mother had, with fewer side effects—all on a diet that allowed 300 *more* calories daily!

Around the same time, I was discovering that very few of my patients were actually adhering to the 520-calorie VLCD. Yes, it worked wonders for people who could follow it religiously, but in truth, compliance was low. Two-thirds of my patients were eating "off the program." The VLCD also had some extremely unpleasant side effects, like nausea, abdominal pain, diarrhea, fatigue, dizziness, and gallstones.

In response to these clinical experiences, I designed a series of studies comparing two groups of patients: those using a shake-based VLCD of 500 calories and those using low-calorie diets of 800 to 1,000 calories daily. In 1994, our team reported that people following the low-calorie diet program and consuming 800 to 1,000 calories daily had lost 20 percent of their initial body weight, while people following the VLCD (500 calories) lost 21 percent of their initial body weight—essentially, the same level of weight loss.[20] Meanwhile, people on the 500-calorie program were experiencing frequent side effects, while people eating the 800-calorie diet were feeling good and had more energy.

Since 1992, we have offered 800-calorie diets to our patients. Tasty and nutritionally balanced entrées soon became available as well, so our patients could choose to use three shakes and two entrées instead of five shakes daily.

In 2000, we began offering nutrition bars to help patients avoid slipping off the program by eating food other than shakes or entrées. At first, I was skeptical that people could use the bars without having too many of them. But while bars are not designed to be meal replacements, they do give variety, and the use of a few bars weekly does not seem to slow weight loss.

# Adding Fruits and Vegetables

Since about 2000, I have been convinced that fruits and vegetables should play a vital role in low-calorie diets. My work (and the work of many other researchers) with dietary fiber for satiety has shown that fruits and vegetables can help dieters feel more full and satisfied. They are also loaded with nutrients and antioxidants, compounds that help protect the body from a variety of chronic diseases.

Including fruits and vegetables in a low-calorie diet also helps the transition back to using whole foods. In short, getting in the habit of including lots of fruits and vegetables in the diet is an important part of learning to maintain weight.

In a recent study published in the *Journal of the American Dietetic Association*, we gave more than two hundred patients the option of choosing either a low-calorie diet based on meal replacements (a combination of shakes and entrées) or the same low-calorie diet plus a minimum of five servings of fruits and vegetables daily. All the patients attended weekly weight-loss meetings, were encouraged to burn at least 2,000 calories a week in physical activity (equivalent to walking two to three miles daily), and kept daily records of their food intake and exercise levels. About two-thirds of patients chose the low-calorie diet alone, while the other third chose the diet plus fruits and vegetables.

The results? The average weight loss for people on the low-calorie diet was 42 pounds in nineteen weeks; the average weight loss for those on the low-calorie diet plus fruits and vegetables was 32 pounds in eighteen weeks—a tolerable difference.[21]

Including a minimum (you can have more if you want) of five servings of fruits and vegetables daily is now part of the weight-loss plan in our clinic. Use of meal replacements, fruits, and vegetables is also a vital part of the Second Phase of the Simple Diet, the health and weight management phase. As long as fruits and vegetables are purchased and prepared without added fat or sugar, they provide a lot of volume, flavor, and interest to meals without adding many extra calories.

## Success with the Simple Diet

With the addition of fruits and vegetables to an 800-calorie diet that is based on meal replacements, we have now arrived at the Simple Diet—what I believe is the most effective, safest, and best solution available for losing a lot of weight quickly and keeping it off. As you can tell from our examples, patients in the program have had great success.

To give you an even broader picture of the success of this program, let me share with you two studies that my colleagues and I recently published, one in the *International Journal of Obesity* and one in the *American Journal of Clinical Nutrition*.

In the first study, we pooled our data from the University of

Kentucky with data from two other similar programs, one in Massachusetts and one in Texas. We all used the same meal replacement products and the same comprehensive approach. At our three centers combined over a seven-year period, eleven hundred people completed a twelve-week initial weight-loss program. Of these eleven hundred people, 268 (24 percent) lost over 100 pounds (not all the patients who started the program needed to lose 100 pounds).

For all the eleven hundred people who completed the twelve-week program, average weight losses over the twelve weeks were 40 pounds for women and 59 pounds for men. For these same people, most of whom continued the program toward goal weight, total weight losses were 68 pounds for women and 94 pounds for men over an average of thirty-nine weeks. Follow-up with these patients at an average of three years later showed that they had maintained about 60 percent of their weight loss.[22]

These are remarkable results.

In the second study, we followed 118 people (sixty-three men and fifty-five women) who lost over 100 pounds while enrolled in the obesity program at the University of Kentucky. The average weight of these people before entering the program was 352 pounds. Almost all participants had obesity-related health conditions, and three-quarters of them were on medications for these conditions.

Average weight loss on the program was 134 pounds in forty-four weeks. About 66 percent of patients on medications for obesity-related health conditions were able to discontinue them, with an average cost-savings of $100 per month. After five years, the average maintained weight loss was 66 pounds. While this shows that some patients regained some of their weight, they still weighed a lot less than when they started.[23] Remember, studies show that most dieters who lose weight regain virtually all of their weight over five years.

With such dramatic improvement to look forward to on the Simple Diet, maybe it's time to get started?

# "I can lose weight safely and consistently by following the Simple Diet."

# Program Essentials and a Fast Start

Now that I've given you some background on the Simple Diet, it's time to get practical. You're getting ready to change your life and there are things to be taken into consideration, some boxes to check before you embark on this incredible journey.

## Talking to Your Doctor

Most weight-loss books include a disclaimer that says something like, "Consult your doctor or other medical professional before beginning this or any other weight-loss program." We have all read plenty of diet books—some of them even written by doctors. But how many of us have actually talked to our own doctors about any of them?

With the Simple Diet, you *must* talk to your doctor. Particularly if you have a medical condition, it is *imperative* that you talk to your doctor before starting this program. Here's why.

My research studies and those of my colleagues have documented that about 97 percent of people with severe obesity have at least one obesity-related condition (and usually more), like high blood pressure, diabetes, or high cholesterol. Seventy-four percent of severely obese people take medications for these conditions. As the individuals I worked with lost excess weight, two out of three were able to discontinue their medications.

But these individuals didn't stop taking the medications on their own; their doctors lowered their doses in *gradual* increments. Eventually, the medications were discontinued. Adjusting medication on your own is dangerous, so you'll need your doctor's help and supervision as you lose weight. In addition, your doctor and medical staff members may be a great source of support and accountability to help you keep with the program.

In chapter 8, I'll explain more about the types of changes you can expect as you lose weight on this program, especially if you have high blood pressure, diabetes, high cholesterol, heart disease, or other obesity-related diseases. I'll provide you with information about how to talk to your doctor. I'll also describe what you and your doctor will need to monitor as you lose weight, and how your doctor may adjust your medications.

## "Why Am I Doing This?"

Take some time to really think about your reasons for losing the extra weight and getting healthy. I expect this is something you've already been thinking about, probably for a long time. In making any sort of commitment, conviction and clarity of intention are key. Everyone will have different reasons, but I see a few recurring themes in this area.

Medical events often can trigger successful weight loss and maintenance. These medical triggers can be the onset of medical conditions, such as high blood pressure, high blood glucose or diabetes, heart disease, or arthritis. An accumulation of medical problems prompted Lance's entry into the program (we'll tell his story later in this chapter). Randy (whose story appears in chapter 10) came in to see me after a heart attack, lost over 100 pounds, and maintained this loss for over twenty years without further heart problems. Andrew lost weight, stopped taking insulin for his diabetes, and was insulin-free for almost twenty years (his story, too, is in chapter 10). I myself have a family history of high blood cholesterol level, high blood pressure, and strokes, so it was fear of having a stroke that first led me to change my own diet. Developing prediabetes further encouraged me to avoid weight gain and be more physically active.

At the VA hospital in Lexington, Kentucky, and in our weight-loss clinic, we have helped hundreds of people get off insulin and stay off insulin for years. These individuals recognized that their weight loss and weight maintenance were essential for them to "avoid the needle."

Maybe your doctor recently told you that your blood pressure was elevated and started you on medicine, or maybe he or she warned you that your blood glucose value would need to be watched, or that your blood triglyceride levels were too high. I find that medical reasons frequently are an initial catalyst to action. But while a health scare may spur you to action, it's far from the only reason you may want to lose weight, and generally I don't find that fear is what keeps an individual on track for the long term.

Having high blood pressure, high blood cholesterol, and prediabetes did not motivate me to lose weight to a health-promoting weight. Rather, it was while attending the baptism of my granddaughter that I decided I wanted to be an important part of her life. This happy thought of joyful living has energized me to become trim and fit. I have five granddaughters, and I want to see each of them reach graduation and other milestones. I want to continue to romp with the children in the ocean on our annual summer vacation. I enjoy travel and want to continue to travel internationally with family and friends. And I love my work and want to continue to make a contribution as long as possible.

Some of the joys my patients share with me that motivate them to achieve a lifetime healthy weight are still being around to see their children and grandchildren reach milestones; being active on the soccer sidelines or shooting baskets with children or grandchildren; climbing stairs to attend games and cultural events; and being able to sit comfortably in theaters, sporting events, or airplanes.

*Angie was a forty-one-year-old third-grade teacher who was anticipating her twentieth wedding anniversary and wanted to lose some weight for her family's trip to Hawaii. With the birth of three children, she had gained 60 pounds since college and wanted to get back to a more healthy weight.*

*Working full-time and chauffeuring three teenagers, she had not found the time (or energy) to seriously address her weight. She was attracted to the program because it did not require a lot of special food preparation and would allow her to follow her diet at school or at soccer practice.*

*At five feet six inches, Angie weighed in at 228 pounds. She started the diet using three shakes, two entrées, and at least five servings of fruits and vegetables daily. This college soccer player had always been active, so she immediately committed to walking daily and hitting the gym three times a week. With this program, she increased her physical activity from less than 1,000 calories per week to 3,600 calories per week. She also increased her diet to three shakes, two or three entrées, one bar, and six to ten servings of fruits and vegetables daily, and lost 15 pounds in four weeks.*

*She lost another 25 pounds in twelve weeks and entered the health and weight management phase to complete her weight loss. For her anniversary trip, she was pleased to weigh in at 168 pounds, a non-obese weight for her large frame.*

People are motivated to lose weight by all different reasons. For Angie, her twentieth wedding anniversary and trip to Hawaii gave her a short-term goal, but what will motivate her to maintain a healthy weight is the ability to more fully enjoy many aspects of her life as well as the extra energy for a demanding schedule. As I shared earlier, I had concerns about my own health that got my attention. But I also have a keen interest in seeing my five granddaughters reach milestones, such as graduations from high school and college. And as a senior adult, I want to continue my extensive national and international travels and stay mentally alert so I can carry on intelligent conversations. These visions motivate me to remain lean and physically fit and to eat healthfully.

The point is that each individual needs to identify for him-

or herself the reasons to lose weight and maintain that weight loss. What motivates you to lose weight now? Start thinking, "I can lose weight because . . ." and make a list of several important aspirations that you have. It is important to write these motives down and read them aloud to yourself. Try to identify a short-term motivation, and also think about the long term and what losing weight will mean to your quality of life for years to come.

## Your Weight-Loss Target

So how much should you weigh ideally?

Many women were at their ideal weight in high school, while men usually achieved their ideal weight around age twenty-one. Everyone should target achieving and maintaining a health-promoting weight that is in the non-obese range. This best-for-health weight is a body mass index (BMI) of less than 25 kg/m². BMI is an internationally accepted measure calculated by dividing the weight in kilograms by the height in meters squared.

Here's how overweight and obesity are defined in terms of BMI:

| | |
|---|---|
| Overweight: | BMI of 25 to 29.9 units |
| Mild obesity: | BMI of 30 to 34.9 units |
| Moderate obesity: | BMI of 35 to 39.9 units |
| Severe obesity: | BMI of more than 40 units |

A BMI chart is located in the appendix (3.1, Body Mass Index Values). Check out what the health-preserving weight is for you. Make sure to use an accurate current weight—the best time to weigh yourself is in the buff before breakfast.

Persons with a large bone structure or frame can carry 10 percent more weight and still be in a healthy zone. To test your frame size, make a bracelet with your right hand around your left wrist. If your right thumb cannot touch your middle finger, you have a large frame and can add 10 percent to your desirable weight. For example, my right thumb overlaps my middle finger when I make this bracelet, so at five feet seven inches tall, my non-overweight goal is 160 pounds. If I had a large frame, I could weigh in at 176 pounds and still be in a healthy range. Of course, athletic individuals who are very well muscled may be "overweight" without having excess body fat. If you consider yourself a trained athlete, you probably should have an estimation of your body fat content at your local YMCA or gym to determine if you have more body fat than is ideal.

Now let's think about weight-loss goals.

The Simple Diet has two phases. The First Phase, the weight-loss phase described in chapters 4 through 9, is very intense, focusing on the Six Keys we'll get to later in this chapter. The Second Phase, the health and weight management phase described in chapter 10, helps you develop a sustainable rhythm to achieve a healthy weight and lifestyle and maintain both for the rest of your life. Ideally, if you have 30 to 50 pounds to lose, you'll lose most of the weight in the First Phase and drop the last few pounds in the Second Phase; if you have 50 to 100 pounds to lose, you'll want to lose 80 percent of the weight in the First Phase and the remainder in the Second Phase. If you have more than 100 pounds to lose, you should try to lose about two-thirds of your weight in the First Phase and the remainder in the Second Phase.

These general recommendations for percentage of weight loss during each phase are based on the experience I have had in helping thousands of individuals achieve and maintain these health-promoting weights over the long haul. I have helped many people, just like you, lose from 30 to 300 pounds and can guide you in this process. One college student lost 270 pounds with my weekly coaching!

To find your weight-loss number, first look at the BMI you calculated earlier. Then think about how much weight you would like to lose and write down what your weight goals are. Was there a particular time in your life when you were at your "perfect weight," when you looked and felt good? How much did you weigh then? Use the BMI chart and ask your doctor to help you decide what your goal should be.

## Will Anything Get in Your Way?

Before I explain the details of the First Phase of the Simple Diet, there's one more thing I'd like you to do: Consider the roadblocks or obstacles you are most likely to encounter. If you take a few minutes now to identify any people or circumstances that could derail your efforts and decide how you will deal with them, you will be far less likely to be stopped in your progress, make excuses, or disappoint yourself.

We all have busy lives, and for many, finding time can be a significant challenge. Can you carve out thirty to sixty minutes daily for physical activity? Or can you create opportunities within your regular routine, ways to do daily tasks that burn more calories? Plan how you will increase your activity.

Also, it's easier to establish and stick with a new routine when you are operating from your home base. Can you find a window of time where you can avoid extended periods of travel for at least three to four weeks to get the Simple Diet down pat?

Are the people around you supportive? It's a good idea to talk with family and friends and get them on board. Share your reasons for wanting to attain a more health-supporting weight, the activities you are looking forward to being able to participate in, or any concerns you may have about the journey. Decide who will be your accountability partner. Plan to check in with that person weekly to let him or her know how you're doing.

Unfortunately, some spouses or other family members may not be supportive. One of my forty-three-year-old patients became a very attractive lady with her weight loss, much to the chagrin of her husband. He did not want his now-attractive wife catching the attention of all the guys in their small town. He consistently worked to torpedo her dieting efforts. For unknown reasons, one mother continually discouraged her son's weight-loss attempts while her husband was very supportive. One mother, a nurse, bought regular Pepsi for herself and Diet Pepsi for her fourteen-year-old, 300-pound son while I was working with him. With some coaching she changed this behavior and stopped bringing regular Pepsi into the home. Whether consciously or unconsciously, family members or friends may have mixed feelings about your following a weight-loss plan. Try to address these concerns before starting the diet. Sometimes having a serious discussion helps people work through their feelings and avoid future problems.

Before you start the program, you may also want to spend a little time making your kitchen diet-friendly. Go through your cupboards and, if possible, get rid of foods that could throw you off track. Reorganize shelves to have your meal replacements front and center in convenient locations you can reach easily. Purchase about a week's worth of meal replacements and a good variety of fresh fruits and vegetables. Keep your food and activity diaries handy. Write down the reasons you want to lose weight, and plan to check in with someone weekly.

# First Phase: Intensive Weight Loss

### ▶ The Six Keys to Intensive Weight Loss

After years of research and experience working with overweight individuals, I have found that there are six crucial keys to rapid, effective, significant weight loss. They may not sound revolutionary or complex enough to work, but I assure you, these six prescriptions, when used consistently, will help you achieve your weight-loss goals.

1. Use at least five meal replacements daily (three shakes, two entrées).
2. Eat at least five servings of fruits and vegetables daily (without added fat or sugar).
3. Add volume and variety (drink a minimum of eight 8-ounce glasses of noncaloric fluids daily; if needed, higher volume of shakes and lower-calorie choices).
4. Build up to burning 2,000 additional calories in physical activity weekly (about two to three miles, or thirty to forty-five minutes, of walking, six days weekly).

5.  Keep daily records of whether you've met or exceeded recommendations (for physical activity and servings of shakes, entrées, fruits, and vegetables).

6.  Be accountable to someone (a family member, friend, or your doctor).

I've studied the effectiveness of these keys in thousands of patients, and I know they work. They will work for you, too. If you follow these keys as I'll describe below, you will see a fast weight loss in the first few weeks of the program, then weeks of steady losses. Although many other factors influence the intake/output calorie balance equation, these six have been shown to be among the most effective for weight loss. They are supported by our research and that of many other clinicians and investigators. For individuals who are really struggling, I'll talk about some additional weight-loss strategies in chapter 9.

I also suggest using self-talk to help you stay focused and positive. Each chapter contains a summary self-talk statement, and more healthy self-talk statements appear in the appendix (3.2, Jump-Start Your Self-Talk).

## Key 1—Use at Least Five Meal Replacements Daily.

Meal replacements—nutritionally and calorically approved preportioned shakes or entrées—take the guesswork out of deciding what or how much to eat. They're a no-stress, no-thought, foolproof way to assure you make the right choices to lose weight quickly. Hundreds of published studies, including many I have been involved with, show that using a highly structured diet that includes meal replacements improves weight loss and weight management compared with diets that have more choices and more room for error. For meal replacements, you'll be using at least three shakes and two entrées daily. Shakes ensure that you get high-quality protein and deliver important fluid intake and satiating volume to your diet. Both fluid and protein play an important role in curbing hunger.

I'll tell you how you can choose the right meal replacements in chapter 4 and offer many options you can purchase at your local grocery or health food store. Although not to be counted as part of your daily meal replacements, you can also eat up to two nutrition bars daily to help satisfy you, provided the bars meet certain criteria I give you in chapter 4.

## Key 2—Eat at Least Five Servings of Fruits and Vegetables Daily.

Adding fruits and vegetables to your meals and snacks gives variety, satisfaction, and high levels of important nutrients without adding a lot of extra calories. And the variety of flavor and texture helps you stay with your plan and keeps you from craving and consuming other higher-calorie foods. More and more clinical research documents the benefits of fruits and vegetables as important adjuncts for weight loss and weight maintenance. I'll give you suggestions for adding fruits and vegetables to your diet in chapter 5. As a general rule, a serving of fruit is one medium piece or one cup, while a serving of vegetable is one cup. Five servings a day of fruits and vegetables will mix things up with your meal replacements while adding great taste and nutrition.

## Key 3—Add Volume and Variety.

The Simple Diet already gives you a lot of volume and variety, with five or more servings of fruits and vegetables combined with filling shakes and entrées. High-volume foods are much more filling than low-volume foods containing the same number of calories. Taking additional steps to add volume and variety to your diet can help even more.

We recommend that you drink at least eight 8-ounce cups of water or noncaloric flavored water daily in addition to the fluid used to mix your shakes. Research clearly shows that drinking a full glass of water before starting a meal decreases food intake and enhances satiety. If you find yourself hungry, you can add more volume to your shakes by using more liquid or ice.

And while all fruits and vegetables are good choices and relatively low in calories compared with French fries, doughnuts, or chips, you can further increase your volume without increasing your calories by choosing the lowest-calorie fruits and vegetables. This is especially helpful if you don't have as much weight to lose or as you near your goal weight. The calorie difference between eating five servings a day of black beans and bananas versus five servings of spinach and strawberries amounts to a weight-loss difference of about a half a pound a week. I'll tell you more about how to add volume and variety to your shakes, entrées, fruits, and vegetables in the next two chapters.

## Key 4—Build Up to Burning 2,000 Additional Calories in Physical Activity Weekly.

Burning 2,000 calories is about the equivalent of walking two to three miles daily or spending thirty to forty-five minutes in active movement daily. I know that, for some of you, this may sound like more than you can do. But if you split up the activity and consistently do three to five minutes of moving around at multiple times during the day, you'll be surprised at how much you can do.

Exercise can be of great benefit to your weight-loss efforts. It also can make you stronger, improve your balance, and improve your mood and sense of well-being. In short, it can improve the quality of your life. For most people, walking is an easy activity to start with, even if you can only walk a few minutes. You'll be surprised how easy it is to add exercise (simply moving your body) if you start slowly and build up gradually. Start with whatever level of activity you are doing now, then try to add ten minutes to that level week one, twenty minutes week two, and so on until you meet your physical activity goal. I'll give you more information about the health and weight management value of regular physical activity and suggestions for how to be more active in chapter 6.

## Key 5—Keep Daily Records of Whether You've Met or Exceeded Recommendations.

Writing down your food intake and physical activity makes you more aware of what you're doing, helps you track your progress, and helps you succeed. Many studies confirm that people who actually write down their food intake and activity levels are more successful at losing weight and keeping it off. There's just something about seeing our efforts and progress in black and white that makes it all more concrete. We think twice about straying from our plan when we write it down. And seeing on paper the success of increasing activity and sticking to your plan will motivate you to keep going.

Keep a daily record of the number of shakes, entrées, and bars you consume, and the number of servings of fruits and vegetables. Also, give yourself credit in your records for staying on the diet (consuming only meal replacements, bars, fruits, and vegetables and no other caloric items), and list the calories you burn in physical activity.

The following tables give daily and weekly summary charts for our program participant Angie. Angie made a little check mark for every shake, entrée, bar, fruit, or vegetable that she consumed, and then totaled the numbers at the end of each day. She exceeded her minimum recommended intake on every single day, had the occasional bar, and still lost four pounds! This is a typical pattern for people starting the diet. In the appendix, you will find a blank template for a daily progress chart that you can photocopy or use as a sample to make your own charts (3.3, Daily Progress Chart). Note that there is a space for the most important self-talk statements you are practicing for that week.

You'll also want to tally your progress week by week. Weekly summaries will help you keep track of your progress. In the appendix is a blank weekly summary chart that you can use or transfer to your own record system (3.4, Weekly Summary Chart). Chapter 7 gives more details on recordkeeping. Be sure to summarize your numbers at the end of each week. Often we find that some of the days with the most meal replacements and fruits and vegetables are days when you feel the best and are worth repeating the next week.

# ANGIE'S DAILY PROGRESS CHART

WEEK OF JAN. 3
STARTING WEIGHT: 223

| DAY | SHAKES | ENTRÉES | FRUITS/ VEGETABLES | BARS | ON THE DIET * | CONSUMED SEFV** | PHYSICAL ACTIVITY |
|---|---|---|---|---|---|---|---|
| Monday | ✓✓✓✓ | ✓✓ | ✓✓✓✓ | ✓ | Y | Y | 200 |
| Tuesday | ✓✓✓✓ | ✓✓ | ✓✓✓✓✓ | | Y | Y | 230 |
| Wednesday | ✓✓✓✓ | ✓✓✓ | ✓✓✓✓✓ | ✓ | Y | Y | 190 |
| Thursday | ✓✓✓✓ | ✓✓ | ✓✓✓✓✓✓ | ✓✓ | Y | Y | 310 |
| Friday | ✓✓✓✓ | ✓✓✓ | ✓✓✓✓✓✓✓ | | Y | Y | 240 |
| Saturday | ✓✓✓✓ | ✓✓✓ | ✓✓✓✓✓✓ | ✓ | Y | Y | 300 |
| Sunday | ✓✓✓ | ✓✓✓ | ✓✓✓✓✓✓✓ | ✓ | Y | Y | 260 |
| Total | 30 | 18 | 49 | 6 | 7 | 7 | 1730 |

*Consumed only meal replacements, bars, fruits, and vegetables, and no other caloric items
**Consumed at least three shakes, two entrées, and five fruits and vegetables (SEFV)

## ANGIE'S WEEKLY SUMMARY CHART

BEGINNING DATE: JAN. 3
BEGINNING WEIGHT: 223

| WEEK | SHAKES | ENTRÉES | FRUITS/ VEGETABLES | BARS | ON THE DIET * | CONSUMED SEFV** | PHYSICAL ACTIVITY | WEIGHT |
|---|---|---|---|---|---|---|---|---|
| 1 | 30 | 18 | 49 | 6 | 7 | 7 | 1730 | 219 |
| 2 | 22 | 18 | 56 | 7 | 7 | 7 | 2200 | 216 |
| 3 | 24 | 15 | 55 | 5 | 6 | 6 | 2530 | 213 |
| 4 | 21 | 20 | 63 | 8 | 7 | 7 | 2840 | 210 |
| 5 | 22 | 17 | 70 | 6 | 7 | 7 | 3220 | 208 |
| 6 | 25 | 18 | 56 | 8 | 6 | 7 | 3610 | 205 |
| 7 | 20 | 17 | 53 | 5 | 7 | 6 | 3520 | 203 |
| 8 | 22 | 19 | 57 | 6 | 7 | 7 | 3810 | 202 |
| 9 | 24 | 15 | 61 | 7 | 7 | 7 | 3620 | 200 |
| 10 | 22 | 18 | 64 | 5 | 7 | 7 | 3510 | 199 |
| 11 | 23 | 19 | 60 | 8 | 6 | 7 | 3830 | 197 |
| 12 | 25 | 17 | 69 | 7 | 6 | 7 | 3610 | 196 |
| 13 | 22 | 15 | 64 | 6 | 7 | 6 | 3520 | 194 |
| 14 | 24 | 17 | 61 | 8 | 7 | 7 | 3650 | 193 |
| 15 | 25 | 21 | 63 | 7 | 7 | 7 | 3590 | 191 |
| 16 | 21 | 17 | 65 | 9 | 6 | 7 | 3720 | 190 |
| 17 | 23 | 18 | 62 | 5 | 7 | 7 | 3590 | 188 |
| 18 | 24 | 16 | 64 | 6 | 7 | 7 | 2870 | 186 |

*Consumed only meal replacements, bars, fruits, and vegetables, and no other caloric items
**Consumed at least three shakes, two entrées, and five fruits and vegetables (SEFV)

## Key 6—Be Accountable to Someone.

Being accountable to someone is helpful—whether it be a family member, close friend, coworker, or member of your health care team. Angie had a very supportive teacher friend who asked her daily about her program. Find someone who is supportive and who will help keep you on track. We'll talk about choosing a health care provider and building support in chapter 8.

# Other Tips for Success

### ▶ Staying Hydrated

Be sure to drink at least eight cups of noncaloric fluid daily *in addition* to the fluid you use to mix with your shakes to stay hydrated. Water is your best choice, but you may also choose seltzer, sparkling water, or diet drink mixes such as Crystal Light. Coffee, tea, and diet sodas are also fine. Some people may find themselves a little dizzy during the first few weeks as they lose weight quickly. Drinking enough fluid as your body adjusts to the lower calorie and sodium content of your diet will help alleviate this problem. After your body adjusts, you'll probably feel better than you have in a long time.

### ▶ Haste to Trim the Waist

Aristotle's famous quote "Well begun is half done" couldn't be more true than when applied to starting the First Phase of the

Simple Diet. A fast start in the first two weeks of the program is one of the best predictors of long-term weight-loss success and is associated with greater total weight loss and maintenance at up to five years of follow-up. I'll help you get off to a fast start, and when you see how good the results feel, you'll want to continue your success.

*Lance had been overweight since college and was very sedentary. He had a long list of problems, including high blood pressure, high blood cholesterol, gout, and sleep apnea. As one medical problem piled on top of another, Lance decided he needed to heed his physician's advice and entered an aggressive weight-loss program.*

*This fifty-eight-year-old attorney was five feet eleven inches tall and weighed in at 369 pounds. As I outlined the plans, Lance was excited and committed himself wholeheartedly to the diet and program. His usual physical activity—walking the bare amount required for daily responsibilities—burned less than 200 calories per week. But he came mentally prepared to do the program and had full support from his wife and children.*

*From the first day on the diet, Lance started walking on the treadmill, sometimes spending an hour per day over several different sessions. He lost 18 pounds in the first week—talk about a fast start! After four weeks on the diet and with a physical activity calorie expenditure exceeding 2,000 calories weekly, Lance had lost 28 pounds. His usual diet included three entrées, three shakes, and one bar daily. By ten weeks, he had lost 52 pounds and his physical activity exceeded 4,400 calories per week. At the six-month mark, he had lost 101 pounds and was doing 8,000 calories of physical activity per week—equivalent to walking forty-five miles per week!*

*Lance now passed his sleep test used to evaluate sleep apnea and no longer needed the CPAP machine. He continued to lose weight using three shakes, three entrées, and about ten servings of fruits and vegetables daily. At a recent visit he was down to 191 pounds, about half his initial weight.*

Using the Six Keys, you can expect to lose 6 to 10 pounds or more within the first few weeks. Getting off to a fast start will motivate you to follow the program and give you momentum as you continue to lose weight. The average woman (initial weight 220 pounds) loses 12 pounds in four weeks, 19 pounds in eight weeks, and 25 more pounds by twelve weeks; the average man (initial weight 267 pounds) loses 22 pounds in four weeks, 31 pounds in eight weeks, and more than 44 pounds in twelve weeks.[24]

Research has shown that the greater your initial weight loss when you start a program, the more likely you are to maintain a significant loss in the long term. In other words, losing weight fast initially is your first step to maintaining a healthy weight and lifestyle over the long term.

Also, the more total weight you lose, the greater the absolute weight loss you're likely to maintain. If you strive to achieve a desirable weight goal because this is a weight you feel good about, you are more likely to sustain this weight loss.

## ▶ Sticking to the Plan

In your initial enthusiasm, you may be tempted to cut out some meal replacements or skip the recommended servings of fruits and vegetables to lose weight even faster, but *don't*. If you skip meal replacements or fruits and vegetables, you will be more likely to go off the plan and eat other higher-calorie foods.

Most people on the Simple Diet find that if they use more shakes and entrées, they do better. If you are having a tough day, plan to have four to five shakes and three to four entrées. The average person I treat can lose weight while eating an average of seven meal replacements and seven servings of fruits and vegetables daily! So do not be hesitant to use more shakes, entrées, fruits, and vegetables if you are having hunger pangs or fatigue, or are getting a slight headache that is slowing down your mental quickness. Chapter 9 provides more guidance for how to stick to the plan if your weight loss is slowing or you are confronting specific challenges.

It's really important to avoid foods that are not on your plan. What we have seen is that the earlier someone goes off the plan, the more likely they are to continue off the plan, and the less weight they are likely to lose. Patients who stayed faithful to the plan for nineteen weeks or more lost over twice the amount of weight that patients who went off the plan the first week did.

Let's look at some data from a study following ninety-three patients who followed a diet similar to the one I am recommending here. Individuals who lost the most weight during the first few weeks of the program were those who stuck to their meal plan and got at least the minimum number of meal replacements plus fruits and vegetables 90 percent or more of the time. Individuals who lost weight slowly during the first few weeks of the program were those who got the minimum number of meal replacements plus fruits and vegetables less than 25 percent of the time. The fast starters lost almost twice as much weight over ten weeks compared with those who did not show as much commitment to their plan and consequently got off to a slow start.[25]

*Brenda was a twenty-four-year-old graduate student in health promotion who was embarrassed that she had gained so much weight in graduate school. At five feet nine inches, she tipped the scales at 204 pounds.*

*Brenda had been a star basketball player who had carried 160 pounds at her peak fitness in college. However, with the stress of graduate school exacerbated by a recent broken engagement, she had stopped running and had been overdoing fast food. Her fasting plasma glucose of 98 mg/dl was on the verge of being in the prediabetic range. Several family members had diabetes, so this got her attention.*

*At our first meeting we talked about her resuming running and doing some weight training. Brenda was a planner. Before she started the Simple Diet, she picked a realistic start date—a time when she had three weeks to get a fast start with no trips or exams to mess with her plans. She was enthusiastic about using three shakes, two entrées, and five servings of fruits and vegetables daily and got off to a very fast start, losing 8.5 pounds in the first week! Brenda followed the shake and entrée regimen religiously and averaged over 3,000 calories per week in physical activity by running twenty-five miles per week and working out.*

*Over eleven weeks, she lost 36 pounds and entered the health and weight management phase, where she dropped another 10 pounds to stabilize at under 160 pounds—her college weight. She kept a spreadsheet of her diet, exercise, weight values, and also favorable changes in her blood pressure, blood glucose, and blood lipids to share with her classmates.*

## ▶ Restaurants, Socializing, and Traveling

Shakes and entrées can be used almost anywhere, and fruits and vegetables are available at almost every place that serves food. If you are invited out to someone's home for dinner, you can have an entrée before leaving home or in the car just before entering their home. Your host or hostess likely will be serving vegetables, and you can discreetly share with him or her that currently you are on a diet. If it is a long evening, you can discreetly have one or two bars that you have carried in a pocket or purse.

Virtually all restaurants and banquets will serve a salad, a vegetable plate, and fruit for dessert. At banquets, I usually alert the server that I am a vegetarian, and they almost always are pleased to accommodate me. I also have had entrées heated up in many fancy restaurants—I hand servers my entrée and a $2 tip for their extra trouble and get a pleasant response.

When we go to dinner parties, I commonly take an entrée and eat vegetables plus my entrée. At potlucks, my wife and I bring cut-up fresh fruit, and I finish my meal with two servings of fruit. When I have luncheon meetings at church or work, I take a double shake in an insulated mug. If fruits and vegetables are not available, the shake will hold me until later. Powdered shake mixes, entrées, and bars pass through screening as carry-on baggage at airports. When I travel, I always have bars available in my computer case, and I often bring an entrée on long flights.

## ▶ Some Last-Minute Considerations

Planning and preparation are essential before you begin the Simple Diet. Before you start, you should try the shakes and entrées to confirm that you can use three shakes and two entrées daily. If you choose to use meal replacement shakes that come in a powdered form, you may want to purchase a blender and set it up in a convenient location. Although most powdered shake mixes dissolve readily in water, having a blender available gives you more options as you whip in ice for extra thickness or try endless combinations of fruit and vegetable shakes and smoothies. (The next two chapters will give you some shake recipes to try.) If your workplace has a kitchen, I also suggest keeping a blender, whisk, or small electric mixer at work. Otherwise, keep stress to a minimum at work using meal replacements that don't need special preparation.

Shop for fruits and vegetables to see what is currently available, and maybe even try some new ones to add variety to your menu. Purchase a full week's supply of shakes, entrées, fruits, and vegetables before you start. Shop for your shakes and entrées at any local grocery or health food store. (You'll find loads of choices in chapter 4 and in the appendix.) Stock up on bars, too. You'll want to buy fruits and vegetables close to when they'll be used so they will be at their freshest and most appealing and you won't have a lot of frustrating spoilage.

Once you finish reading more about the Six Keys to Intensive Weight Loss outlined in chapters 4 through 8, you'll be well on your way to weight-loss success!

## ▶ Getting in at Least the Minimum

To get in the recommended minimum of three shakes, two entrées, and five fruits and vegetables daily, you can either double up two meal replacements at some meals (for example, an entrée and a shake), or you can space your meal replacements, fruits, and vegetables throughout the day to keep you from getting hungry.

Try having a meal replacement shake or entrée for breakfast, lunch, and dinner, then in between have two more meal replacements for snacks. Add your five servings of plain fruits and vegetables to meals and snacks, and you've met the daily minimum. Try a fruit smoothie, for example, or add cooked vegetables to your entrées. It may seem like you are eating all the time, but if you spread out your food intake to three meals and two or three snacks daily, you'll be surprised how satisfied you feel. You may even find it helpful to plan out the day's menus ahead of time. See the sample menu below.

## Sample Menu

**Breakfast**  ▶ Strawberry shake (Special K) blended with 1 banana

**Morning Snack**  ▶ 1 cup cantaloupe

**Lunch**  ▶ Ravioli Florentine (Smart Ones) (or entrée of choice), 1 cup roasted mushrooms, tomatoes, and zucchini

| Afternoon Snack | ▶ Rich Chocolate Royale shake (Slim-Fast) |
| Dinner | ▶ Roasted Chicken Marsala (Healthy Choice) (or entrée of choice), 1 cup steamed carrots, 1 cup steamed snap peas |
| Evening Snack | ▶ Creamy Eggnog (see recipe on page 60) |

Still feel hungry? Go ahead and have an extra meal replacement or more fruits and vegetables. It's hard to overeat with these foods, and having the extra servings of meal replacements or fruits and vegetables will keep you from going off your plan. You can also have up to two high-protein bars daily if you still feel hungry (see chapter 4 and the appendix for plan-friendly bars).

I also recommend that everyone on the Simple Diet take a low-dose multivitamin and mineral supplement daily to assure adequate intake of important nutrients. You can use a modest amount of sugar-free gum or candy if you want to, but be aware that these products contain sugar alcohols that in large quantities can give you gas, cramping, and diarrhea.

Remember, people who stay on the plan, even if they use more than the minimum number of meal replacements, fruits, and vegetables, are the ones who lose the most weight. Research with over five hundred individuals has shown that people who followed the Six Keys and ate only meal replacements, fruits, and vegetables lost more than three times as much weight as people who used fewer meal replacements but may have gone off the program.

When you eat food that is not on the diet, you are likely consuming more calories and also greatly increasing the likelihood that you will discontinue the diet before you reach your health-promoting weight goal.

# Making Room for the Second Phase

The First Phase, the intensive weight-loss phase of the Simple Diet, is time-limited and highly structured, and focuses your attention on being on the diet every day, with no other grocery foods except fruits and vegetables to achieve aggressive, consistent weight loss. How long you stay in the First Phase depends on your current weight and your weight-loss goals.

In the Second Phase, the health and weight management phase, you'll focus on practicing healthy lifestyle habits and using meal replacements along with a variety of other healthy foods to sustain gradual weight loss or long-term health and weight management. As my good friend and fellow weight-loss physician Dr. Jim Early says, "In the First Phase, you are the student and we serve as educators, while in the Second Phase, you are the player and we are the coaches."

The goal of this book is to help you be healthy players for life. We'll talk more about the Second Phase in chapter 10.

"I can commit to improving my health and enjoying life more by meeting my diet, exercise, and recordkeeping goals."

# Meal Replacements: Shakes, Entrées— and Success

Following the Simple Diet is really quite easy. At the beginning, you'll be using three shakes and two entrées daily, along with at least five servings of fruits and vegetables. The meal replacements we recommend are nutritionally balanced and take any guesswork out of deciding what to eat. I've researched many types of meal replacements and can tell you that finding a variety of appropriate shakes and entrées will be easy. In this chapter (and in greater detail in the appendix), you'll find Simple Diet–approved shakes and entrées from Banquet, Equate, GNC, Healthy Choice, Lean Cuisine, Michelina's, Revival Soy, Slim-Fast, Slim-Rite, Smart Ones, Special K, and more!

# What Are My Meal Replacement Choices?

Although many commercially available meal replacement products meet our careful nutritional and calorie guidelines, not *all* replacements are created equal. The table below lists the criteria we have established to determine whether a given meal replacement product meets acceptable nutrition guidelines for calorie, protein, and fat content. Using these guidelines, you can quickly assess any shake on the grocery shelves or entrée in the supermarket freezer.

| | CALORIES (KCAL) | | PROTEIN (GRAMS) | | FAT (GRAMS) | |
|---|---|---|---|---|---|---|
| | Minimum | Maximum | Minimum | Maximum | Minimum | Maximum |
| **Shakes** | 100 | 200 | 10 | 26 | 0 | 6 |
| **Entrées** | 140 | 300 | 10 | 25 | 0 | 9 |
| **Soups** | 100 | 200 | 10 | 20 | 0 | 6 |
| **Bars** | 100 | 200 | 6 | 20 | 0 | 5 |

To be suitable for the Simple Diet, shakes and entrées need to give you the maximum bang for your calorie buck. This means that they should provide at least 10 grams of protein. Soups that meet this important 10 grams of protein criterion can count as a shake and also be used to add variety. Nutrition bars are not meal replacements, but they give you some flexibility. I'll provide more details on that a little later.

Many shakes comply with our criteria and can provide complete nutrition. Shakes are filling because of their high volume, yet they have low calorie levels, and can be made with many different noncaloric flavorings into blasts, blizzards, coladas, delights, dreams, floats, mousses, puddings, smoothies, and other personal favorites. I enjoy having a bottle of Special K Milk Chocolate Protein Shake midmorning and then having a packet of Revival Soy Vanilla Pleasure blended with 16 ounces of diet root beer in the midafternoon. We recommend having at least three shakes daily. Below are just some of the many shakes that meet our criteria; Appendix 4.1, Recommended Shakes, gives a more complete list of suitable shakes.

- Blueberry Blush (Revival Soy)
- Cappuccino Delight (Slim-Fast)
- Creamy Milk Chocolate (Slim-Rite)
- French Vanilla (Slim-Rite)
- Just Peachy! (Revival Soy)
- Rich Chocolate Royale (Slim-Fast)
- Strawberries N' Cream (Slim-Fast)
- Strawberry (Special K)
- Vanilla Bean (GNC)

People who don't have as much weight to lose (those who weigh less than 180 pounds) and people who have been on the Simple Diet for a while and are approaching their goal weight may find adding extra volume to their shakes helps satisfy them and allows them to maintain a lower calorie intake, boosting weight loss. (We'll talk more about this strategy in chapter 9.) If you need more volume, either for satiety or because your weight loss is slowing, you can make your shakes more filling by adding more ice or zero-calorie liquids, like diet soda or coffee, in addition to water to give you twice the volume for equal calories. Adding sugar-free gelatin can add texture and volume to your shakes, too. I enjoy making a double vanilla shake with 12 ounces of diet root beer, 8 ounces of water, a half packet of sugar-free gelatin, and four ice cubes. Another option is to replace root beer with water and add 1 tablespoon of sugar-free dark cocoa. As outlined in chapter 5, you can add fruit to make tasty smoothies or frappes. Here are just a few shake recipes to enjoy.

You can buy many shakes in powder form or in ready-to-drink liquid form. Follow package directions for mixing powdered shakes, but here are general basic directions.

1. Pour about 6 oz. of cold water into a blender.
2. Add one serving of shake mix and any flavorings (see page 60 for other flavoring ideas). Blend on lowest speed.
3. Add four ice cubes, one at a time, making sure to replace blender cover after each ice cube, and blend briefly.
4. Blend on low speed for 1–1½ minutes, until shake is smooth.
5. Blend on high speed for another 10 seconds for an extra-creamy shake.

You can combine fruit with your shake to make a delicious fruit smoothie:

# Strawberry-Kiwi Smoothie

¾ cup water

1 serving vanilla-flavored powdered shake mix

1 cup frozen strawberries

½ cup fresh kiwi, peeled

artificial sweetener, if desired

# Raspberry Smoothie

¾ cup diet ginger ale

1 serving vanilla-flavored powdered shake mix

1 cup frozen raspberries

Or you can add different flavorings to your shake to add some variety to your diet:

# Banana Colada

¾ cup water

1 serving vanilla-flavored powdered shake mix

¼ tsp. banana extract

¼ tsp. rum extract

⅛ tsp. cinnamon

# Chocolate Almond Surprise

¾ cup water

1 serving chocolate-flavored powdered shake mix

¼ tsp. almond extract

## Creamy Eggnog

¾ **cup water**

**1 serving vanilla-flavored powdered shake mix**

⅛ **tsp. vanilla extract**

⅛ **tsp. rum or brandy extract**

⅛ **tsp. ground nutmeg**

## Mocha Cooler

¾ **cup water**

**1 serving chocolate-flavored powdered shake mix**

**1 tsp. instant coffee**

Other flavoring options include:

- Almond extract, ¼ tsp.
- Banana extract, ¼ tsp.
- Cinnamon, dash or ⅛ tsp.
- Cocoa, 1 tsp.
- Coconut extract, ¼ tsp.
- Coffee, instant (caffeinated or decaffeinated), 1 tsp.
- Gelatin mix, sugar-free, flavor of your choice, ½ packet
- Instant pudding mix, sugar-free/fat-free, flavor of your choice, 1 tbsp.
- Maple extract, 1 tsp.
- Nutmeg, ¼ tsp.
- Pumpkin pie spice, 1 tsp.
- Rum extract, ¼ tsp.
- Vanilla extract, ⅛ tsp.

You can also make tasty soda floats using your favorite diet soda (cream, ginger ale, orange, cola, root beer, etc.):

1. Add 12 oz. of cold soda to blender.
2. Begin mixing at lowest speed.
3. While blender is on, add shake mix.
4. While blender is going, add four ice cubes, one at a time.
5. Continue mixing on lowest speed for 1½ minutes until ice is thoroughly blended and shake is smooth.

For many years, it was our protocol to treat obese patients with very-low-calorie diets of five or more shakes per day and nothing else (see chapter 2). Then, under research conditions, we tested the addition of entrées to the nutrition plan. We found that using three shakes and two entrées was equally effective and less restrictive than using only shakes and resulted in greater patient adherence and satisfaction with far fewer side effects.

For the last fifteen years, given a choice, most people in the clinic program have elected to use entrées in addition to shakes. This adds a few more calories, but the variety helps people stay on the diet much better. We recommend eating at least two entrées daily and have identified more than two hundred that meet our nutrition guidelines of providing 140 to 300 calories, 10 to 25 grams of protein, and 0 to 9 grams of fat. Below are some examples of entrées that meet these guidelines, and Appendix 4.2, Recommended Entrées, provides a more exhaustive list. You'll find a range of choices, including beef, chicken, fish, pasta, pizza, pork, and turkey entrées. Most vendors have websites, and many will ship to your home.

- Chicken Marsala (Smart Ones)
- Chicken Romano Fresca (Healthy Choice)
- Chicken Nuggets with Fries (Banquet)
- Fettuccine Alfredo with Broccoli (Michelina's)
- Four Cheese Cannelloni (Lean Cuisine)
- Garlic Roasted Shrimp (Healthy Choice)
- Golden Roasted Turkey Breast (Healthy Choice)
- Orange Chicken (Lean Cuisine)
- Pasta Primavera (Smart Ones)
- Ravioli Florentine (Smart Ones)
- Salisbury Steak (Healthy Choice)
- Swedish Meatballs with Pasta (Lean Cuisine)
- Three Cheese Ravioli (Weight Watchers)

When using a soup as a meal replacement, count it as a shake. Soup can be used as is, used as a sauce for an entrée, or mixed with an entrée to make a thicker soup, stew, casserole, or goulash. For instance, adding a chicken entrée such as Lean Cuisine Chicken and Vegetables to your already prepared hot chicken soup makes a heartier and delicious dish that counts as one shake and one entrée in your daily plan. We only identified the few soups listed below that come in a single serving and meet our recommendations. All are from Healthy Choice. You can also find more options in the appendix (4.4, Recommended Soups). If you are a soup-lover, you can find many acceptable soups by visiting the websites of commercial brands. Make sure to pay attention to serving size. Many cans of soups contain two servings.

- Healthy Choice Bean & Ham
- Healthy Choice Chicken Tortilla

- Healthy Choice Italian Style Wedding
- Healthy Choice Split Pea & Ham
- Healthy Choice Steak & Noodle
- Healthy Choice Vegetable Beef

New products enter the market continually, so I am confident that you will be able to find an array of foods that meet your needs for taste and variety. And purchasing shakes and entrées could not be easier. With so many choices, you can get yours in any grocery store in the country—even in a local convenience store.

Nutrition bars are convenient and can contribute to your success. However, we consider bars only for emergency use, when entrées or shakes are not available, or when time does not allow making a shake. *We do not consider bars to be meal replacements.* Bars often do not contain adequate protein to count as a meal replacement, and because they usually provide about 100 or more calories per ounce (as compared with 30 calories per ounce for entrées and 10 to 20 calories per ounce for shakes), they are much less satisfying and filling. We recommend that you do not use more than seven bars per week. Below is a list of bars that meet our nutrition criteria, but remember to use them judiciously. More bars are listed in Appendix 4.3, Recommended Bars.

- Berry Almond (Luna)
- Blueberry Flax & Soy (Optimum)
- Chocolate Peanut Butter (Balance)
- Honey Almond Flax (Kashi)
- LemonZest (Luna)
- Peanut Butter Cookie Dough (Zone)

- Strawberry Shortcake (Pure Protein)
- Trail Mix (Kashi)
- Vanilla Zest (GNC)
- Yogurt Honey Peanut (Balance)

# Aren't Meal Replacements Expensive?

Currently, the average U.S. adult weighs about 180 pounds and spends about $113 per week on food eaten at home and away from home.[26] Over the years, many individuals who came to see me for weight management weighed somewhere in the area of 240 pounds, or about 33 percent more than average. Let's estimate that the average obese person, at 240 pounds, consumes 20 percent more food than the average U.S. adult. This conservative estimate suggests that the 240-pound individual probably spends about $136 per week for food.

Meal replacement entrées from the grocery store cost from $0.88 (yes, that's right—as this was written, I purchased Banquet entrées at my Walmart for $0.88) to $4.00, and a nice selection of meal replacements is available for about $2.00 each when they are on sale (and it seems that one brand or another is on sale every week!). At this price, fourteen meal replacements would cost about $28 for the week. Shakes cost in the range of $0.75 to $1.25 per shake, or about $21 for a week of shakes. Fruits and vegetables, as discussed in chapter 5, cost about $0.30 per serving, or less than $12 per week.

Thus, the frugal shopper can purchase all of the food recommended for the Simple Diet for $61 per week ($28 + $21 + $12), saving up to $75 per week in food costs while on the Simple Diet!

# Why Are Meal Replacements So Effective in Promoting Weight Loss?

I have developed hundreds of recipes, from my early research days to later recipes included in books, newsletters, and our website. To determine accurate nutrition information for these recipes, I had to weigh and measure *everything*. Lacking the time and interest to do this as we prepare our meals each day, most people will take shortcuts, and before they know it will find themselves eating off the diet.

But prepackaged shakes and entrées already contain the right amount of calories, protein, fat, and other nutrients, so they're a quick and easy way for individuals with busy lifestyles to assure adequate nutrient intake, satisfying volume, and low enough calories for fast weight loss. Angie, the busy mother and teacher featured in the last chapter, loved the decision-free aspect of the plan. She could, without thinking, grab an entrée box and a couple packets of shakes as she rushed out of the house in the morning, knowing she could supplement with a salad at school and have a filling lunch.

Even when not dieting, many people do not get enough of the right nutrients in the food they eat. Any time you then put yourself on a calorie-reduced diet, it's even more important that you are getting adequate nutrition to avoid mineral and vitamin deficiencies. And, as we have learned from recent research, protein is a very important component of a diet because it is the most satiating (filling) nutrient you can eat. Fruits and vegetables provide variety, some calories and nutrients, and protective phytochemicals, but don't include the range of nutrients provided in the recommended shakes and entrées. It's your meal replacements that are keys to good nutrition and a high protein intake during the First Phase.

And it's your meal replacements that are helping you to cut those calories effortlessly. Small dietary changes can have big consequences over time. Consider two possible breakfasts you could choose: a piece of fruit plus either a large purchased muffin at 500 calories, or a shake that meets your nutritional criteria at 100 calories. If you chose the shake over the muffin even just twice a week for a year, the 800 saved calories per week would be enough to result in a 12-pound weight loss in a year!

Simply put, using proportioned and nutritionally balanced shakes and entrées reduces decision making and hassle. For the busy individual, it's really easier to stick to the diet than to stray! Also, people lose more weight more quickly on the Simple Diet than with any other strategy that has been tested—building confidence and satisfaction. Experiencing this level of success early on in the diet tends to raise the commitment and compliance levels, leading to even greater success.

## How Does a Meal Replacement–Based Diet Stack Up Against Other Popular Plans?

Meal replacements—including both shakes and entrées—are a very effective tool for weight loss and long-term health and weight management. We have used meal replacements in our research and clinical practice for twenty years and have documented that this approach is more effective than any other lifestyle approach. Dr. Chris Gardner and his associates at Stanford

University School of Medicine did a carefully controlled study of three of the most popular diets that do not use meal replacements (the Atkins diet, the Ornish diet, and the Zone diet) in overweight and obese individuals with a BMI ranging from 27 to 40.[27] We compared results with these three diets to results in our own recently published study of overweight and obese individuals in a similar weight range who used a diet that includes meal replacements, fruits, and vegetables.[28]

Two months after starting the diet, participants had lost the following amounts of weight: on the Zone diet, 4.6 pounds; on the Ornish diet, 5.3 pounds; on the Atkins diet, 9.5 pounds; and on the Simple Diet, 18.7 pounds. Individuals using meal replacements lost more than three times as much weight as individuals on the Zone or Ornish diets and twice as much weight as individuals on the Atkins diet. Weight losses of 18 to 24 pounds are typical for our patients during the First Phase of the Simple Diet. Further, our study did not include severely obese individuals, who usually lose substantially more weight than mild or moderately obese individuals.

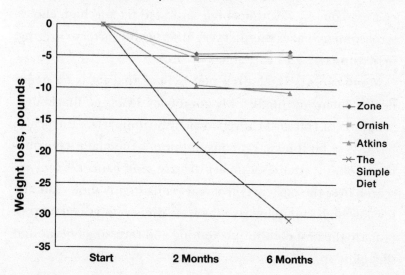

Differences in weight-loss results on the different diets were even more striking as time went on. Six months after starting the diet, participants had lost and/or maintained the following amounts of weight: on the Zone diet, 4.2 pounds; on the Ornish diet, 4.8 pounds; on the Atkins diet, 10.6 pounds; and a diet using three shakes and two entrées, 30.6 pounds. At six months, our patients using meal replacements had lost about six times more weight than individuals on the Ornish or Zone diets and three times more than individuals on the Atkins diet. Further, participants in our study entered the Second Phase of the program at sixteen weeks and continued to lose weight nicely (a half pound weekly) during this phase. These comparisons show the effectiveness of including meal replacements in the weight-loss plan.

Although the Atkins diet has been extremely popular and highly promoted, research shows that our approach using meal replacements for weight loss and long-term health and weight management is more effective than the Atkins diet. A further caution: The high fat content of the Atkins diet (55 percent of energy) combined with its high saturated fat and high cholesterol content makes this diet very atherogenic (artery-clogging, increasing risk for heart attack or stroke).

Many experts (including me) believe that fat is *the* major health enemy in the diet. My good friend George Blackburn, MD, PhD, at Harvard University plainly summarizes the health hazards of fat intake: Fat consumption is the major contributor to obesity, diabetes, heart disease, and cancer.[29] Our research over the past forty-five years consistently shows that the low-fat, high–complex carbohydrate diets with adequate protein are the best diets for preventing and reversing obesity and diabetes.

# Adding Volume and Variety

*Denise, a fifty-six-year-old grandmother who weighed in at 207 pounds, took medications for high blood pressure, high cholesterol, and acid reflux. She retired from a retail sales position to spend more time with her three grandchildren. With her family history of heart attacks, she decided to get serious about her health so she could participate in her grandchildren's upcoming graduations and other milestones.*

*Being an excellent cook, Denise knew how to get creative with the shakes, entrées, fruits, and vegetables, developing her own recipes that her whole family could enjoy. She purchased twice as many entrées and shakes as she needed for her own diet so that she could share them with her supportive husband and busy daughter and son-in-law, as well as her grandchildren. As part of her commitment to walk three miles daily, she regularly walked to several different farmers' markets, where she gathered choice fresh fruits and vegetables.*

*With the casseroles and vegetable recipes she developed, not to mention her tasty combinations of various entrées, Denise could write an entire cookbook. Her grandchildren preferred "Mamaw's smoothies" to fast-food shakes and ice cream.*

*At a large-framed five feet one inch, Denise had a goal weight of 135 pounds. Over the course of twenty-four weeks, she lost 67 pounds and jettisoned all of her prescription medications. While stopping her medications, her blood pressure dropped from 136/84 to 112/68 mm Hg, her LDL cholesterol (the bad kind) from 120 to 73 mg/dl, and her glucose from a prediabetic level of 110 to 78 mg/dl.*

*Denise continued to lose weight in the Second Phase of the program, the health and weight management phase. One year after completing the First Phase, the intensive weight-loss phase, Denise was still enjoying entrées and shakes combined with a low-fat diet and weighed in at 140 pounds.*

Denise had the time to be creative, adding her own gourmet twists to her Simple Diet choices that both she and her family enjoyed. The basic ingredients are varied enough that our patients have found the diet very acceptable, using the shakes, entrées, fruits, and vegetables in many different ways. You, too, will find the Simple Diet both easy to follow and fun to adapt to your own preferences as you lose weight.

Hundreds of available meal replacements, including shakes, entrées, and soups, meet our nutritional guidelines. You can add endless variety by combining two meal replacements to make tasty casseroles or, as you'll see in the next chapter, by combining a meal replacement with fruits and vegetables. There are so many products that meet our criteria, you'll find thousands of delicious combinations.

## How *Should* I Use Bars?

The judicious use of bars has been a very useful addition to our diet. However, a word of caution: I can consume three 1.5-ounce bars in fifteen minutes, having inhaled 480 calories in a volume of only 4.5 ounces and saddling me with over 100 calories per ounce. Instead, I could have eaten an entrée at 240 calories in 8 ounces—half the calories in twice the volume—adding only 30 calories per ounce, leaving me more satisfied and allowing me to go longer before feeling hungry again.

Although bars are not intended to substitute for meal replacements, they can be used tactically to enhance your weight loss by keeping you from eating food that is not included on the Simple Diet. When I travel, I always carry several bars in my computer bag. When I go out to eat at a friend's house or restaurant, I usually have a bar in my jacket pocket in case I am only able to eat the vegetables or fruit provided, which does not sustain me for four hours of conversation. However, here's a cautionary tale: One of my patients ate an average of fifty bars per week for a twelve-week period. This intelligent attorney wondered why she was not losing weight, because she only ate foods that were recommended and consumed at least three shakes and two entrées per day! The typical person we treat does fine consuming less than one bar per day on average.

# Your Most Effective Tool for Weight Loss

Use of meal replacements is *the* most effective tool for successful weight loss, and the Simple Diet program is *the* most successful nonsurgical weight-loss plan you can try. This intervention is more than three times as effective as many popular diets (such as the Ornish diet) and twice as effective as most commercial programs (such as Jenny Craig).

You have many diet plans to choose from. However, we are confident that no other plan offers the variety, convenience, affordability, and effectiveness of the Simple Diet. With this plan, you *will* lose weight and improve your health.

"I can set a health-maintaining weight goal and I have the determination to achieve that goal by consuming at least three shakes, two entrées, and five servings of fruits and vegetables daily."

# Fruits and Vegetables: Adding Volume and Variety

J eff, a fifty-three-year-old manager in a fire department, came to see me when he learned that one of his colleagues had been able to discontinue insulin treatment while under my care. Jeff had heart disease, had had two heart stents inserted six months previously, and wanted to lose weight to improve his health and decrease his need for medication.

In addition to heart disease, he had diabetes and was taking sixty units of insulin daily and three pills for his diabetes. He had high blood pressure and took two blood pressure medications. He also had high blood cholesterol and was on one pill daily to lower it. At five feet nine inches tall and with a weight of 249 pounds, Jeff was in the moderately obese category.

I saw Jeff in the clinic, and we developed a treatment program for him to follow at home. After a long discussion,

*Jeff indicated that he could consume six to eight servings of vegetables daily. We agreed on the following plan: He would have a shake and fresh fruit for breakfast; a midmorning shake; a salad, an entrée of his choice, and fruit for lunch; an entrée, two generous servings of vegetables, and two servings of fruit for dinner; and a shake in the evening. He committed to follow the Simple Diet and agreed to increase his walking from zero to forty minutes daily.*

*Jeff monitored his blood glucose carefully, and we agreed to decrease his insulin dose to half the current dose and stop one of his diabetes pills. Jeff left the office in a very upbeat mood and followed the plan to a T. In two weeks, he called me and reviewed his blood glucose records. We then reduced his insulin dose to twenty units per day.*

*In four weeks, Jeff bounded into the office, down 20 pounds and having kept good food, exercise, and blood glucose records. He was consuming at least eight servings of fruits and vegetables daily. Based on his blood glucose and blood pressure values, we stopped his insulin completely, a second diabetes pill, and one blood pressure medication.*

*Over the next three months, I saw Jeff monthly, we exchanged the occasional e-mail, and he continued to do well. On his fifth visit, after sixteen weeks, Jeff was down 51 pounds and was off insulin and all his medications. He was walking three miles daily and using the weight machines at work. Jeff was very excited because, at 199 pounds, he was at his lowest weight since high school. He suggested that he was more physically fit than many of the firemen he supervised. He was a walking billboard for the treatment program and never hesitated to brag about his success and the effectiveness of the treatment approach.*

Fruits and vegetables are among the healthiest foods you can eat and serve your family. They have a very important role in weight loss, in health and weight management, and in reducing risk for heart disease, stroke, diabetes, and some cancers. According to Yale University's Overall Nutritional Quality Index, fruits and vegetables make up 95 percent of the healthiest foods (foods rated 90 to 100 out of 100 for several nutritional quality variables).

For weight loss, fruits and vegetables add variety and volume to your diet. The huge variety of fruits and vegetables available keeps your diet interesting and gives you a myriad of options to combine with shakes and entrées. Not only are fruits and vegetables nutritious in their own right, but they also displace other higher-calorie foods that you might otherwise eat, keeping your calorie intake low. In this chapter, I will share with you how to include fruits and vegetables in the Simple Diet.

When Jeff came to see me in our university clinic, he chose not to enroll in the program, but elected to follow the Simple Diet with my coaching. His story illustrates both the health benefits of weight loss and the value of consuming generous amounts of fruits and vegetables.

Jeff consumed between six and ten servings of fruits and vegetables daily. In the first month, Jeff lost 20 pounds and cut his insulin dose to one-third of initial values. After two months, with Jeff down 34 pounds, we stopped his insulin and all medications for high blood pressure and blood cholesterol levels. His blood glucose and blood pressure returned to the normal range, and he was now off insulin and required none of his six original medications. His pharmacy bill dropped from $325 to $25 per month, and he only had to prick his finger for blood glucose measurements once daily rather than four times daily. You can see why Jeff was so thrilled.

Jeff is representative of the many patients I have supervised using meal replacements enhanced with fruits and vegetables. A generous intake of fruits and vegetables will be extremely beneficial in your First Phase (intensive weight loss), in your Second Phase (health and weight management), and thereafter in a healthy diet for life. The average individual who commits to the Simple Diet and follows it for at least eight weeks loses 35 pounds in fifteen weeks. The 20 percent of people who are the least successful when following the program lose 19 pounds in twelve weeks—that's not terrible. But maybe you'd like to be like the 20 percent of people who follow the Simple Diet most diligently and lose 62 pounds in eighteen weeks![30]

What sets this 20 percent of people who lose the most weight apart from the rest? Like everyone on the Simple Diet, they practice the Six Keys outlined in chapter 3, averaging at least three shakes and two entrées daily, staying on the diet faithfully, using occasional bars, and logging more than 2,000 calories per week in physical activity. But they also eat *over six fruits and vegetables per day*. Emphasizing fruits and vegetables plays a key role in keeping you feeling satisfied and on the diet, leading to successful weight loss.

# Choosing Your Fruits and Vegetables

On the Simple Diet, you can choose any fresh, frozen, or canned fruit or vegetable without added fat or sugar (and prepared and served with no added fat or sugar). These provide an average of only about 50 calories in a 4-ounce serving. At the higher end of the calorie spectrum, you'll find avocados and garbanzo beans at 47 and 51 calories per ounce, respectively (or 125 and 157 calories per ½-cup serving). At the lower end of the spectrum you'll find watermelon and celery, at 7 and 4 calories per ounce, respectively (or 42 and 20 calories per one-cup serving). When eating a wide variety of fruits and vegetables, it all averages out to about 12.5 calories per ounce.

One caveat: We don't recommend dried fruit for the Simple Diet. Dried fruit averages over 70 calories per ounce—a high calorie level for a small volume of food that can be wolfed down quickly and is not very filling or satisfying. On the Simple Diet, we emphasize foods that are low in calories and high in volume (the actual space a food takes up in your stomach), helping you feel full and satisfied.

So does it matter if you choose fresh, frozen, or canned fruits and vegetables? Although fresh fruits and vegetables contain the highest levels of nutrients and health-promoting antioxidants (substances that help protect your body cells from damage), frozen fruits and vegetables are processed just hours after picking, before they have time to lose nutritional value, and are a very close second to fresh. Even canned fruits and vegetables, while having lost just a small percentage of their nutritive value in the heating process, are still packed with nutrients and are excellent choices as compared with doughnuts or candy bars. Calorie-wise, fresh, frozen, and canned are all the same.

If you use frozen or canned fruits and vegetables, read labels and be sure you buy ones with no added sugar or fat. Avoid fruits packed in syrup or vegetables frozen in a butter or cheese sauce. If I use canned fruit, I rinse the fruit to get rid of extra sugar and then sprinkle a packet of Splenda on it to add sweetness. I also rinse canned vegetables to get rid of some of the extra salt and then often sprinkle with Mrs. Dash seasonings. For the budget shopper, canned fruits and vegetables are, on average, cheaper than other forms and have a very long shelf life. But whether shopping at an upscale market or a discount store, I find that fruits and vegetables cost an average of about $0.35 per serving. Better yet, walk to your local farmer's market, save some money, and get a variety of fresh local vegetables bursting with flavor. Either way, you can fill your shopping basket and enjoy.

All fruits and vegetables deliver high nutrition quality. The only food that comes close to the nutritional quality of fruits and vegetables is skim milk, at 60 calories per 8 ounces, or 7.5 calories per ounce. Consider some other possible food choices:

- bread, 70 calories per ounce
- hamburger, 75 calories per ounce
- cake, 110 calories per ounce
- doughnut, 110 calories per ounce
- cheese, 120 calories per ounce
- candy bar, 135 calories per ounce
- potato chips, 160 calories per ounce
- almonds, 170 calories per ounce

All of these items, from breads to almonds, are *high energy dense*, meaning they deliver lots of calories per ounce. The excellent research of Dr. Barbara Rolls and others clearly shows that high energy-dense foods contribute to weight gain and should be avoided during weight loss and management efforts. So compared with other food choices we could be making, *any* fruit or vegetable is always a good choice.

Yes, potatoes have more calories than celery. At 27 calories per ounce, potatoes are in the higher calorie range for vegetables, but potato chips still have *six times* more calories per ounce than baked potatoes. At this stage of intensive weight loss with drastic calorie reductions in other areas, the small difference in calories from potatoes versus celery will not matter much for most people.

It *is* more important to take the small differences into account when you don't have as much weight to lose, if your weight loss is slowing, or if you are approaching your goal weight. Then you may find it helpful to choose lower-calorie fruits and vegetables. Recently, I counseled a lady who was losing weight slowly that there were lots of other fruit and vegetable options besides her favorites, which appeared to be bananas and potatoes!

In the appendix, you will find lists of low-, moderate-, and high-calorie fruits (5.1, Low-, Moderate-, and High-Calorie Classification of Fruits) and vegetables (5.2, Low-, Moderate-, and High-Calorie Classification of Vegetables). For now, you don't need to worry about these lists; just focus on getting at least five servings a day of any fruits and vegetables. But as we'll discuss more in chapter 9, if you weigh less than 180 pounds, if your weight loss is slowing, or when you are nearing your goal weight, you may want to choose the lowest of the already low-calorie fruits and vegetables.

Later on, as you transition to the Second Phase of the Simple Diet, you will need to become more aware of calories from all sources of foods in addition to those from fruits and vegetables. We will introduce you to the Green Light Calorie Guide in chapter 10. For now, we will share that all fruits and vegetables are in the "green" for "go ahead and eat all you want" category, meaning that they are high in nutrition and low in calories.

# What about Fruit and Vegetable Juices?

Although fruit and vegetable juices are certainly better than many other beverage choices, we do not recommend juices on the Simple Diet. Many juices contain added sugar. Even if they don't, one cup of apple juice contains about 120 calories and takes ten seconds to drink. One medium apple contains about 80 calories and takes ten minutes to eat.

Eating whole fruits and vegetables is much more satiating than drinking juice. Whole fruits and vegetables provide more volume for fewer calories, take longer to consume, and satisfy the need to chew something substantial. In addition, whole fruits and vegetables contain dietary fiber, an indigestible portion of food that has many health benefits, as we'll talk about in chapter 12.

# What Counts as a Serving?

Except for very dense fruits like avocados, bananas, or cherries, one serving of fruit is one medium piece of fruit or one cup of sliced fruit or berries. For bananas, one serving is half of a banana. For cherries and avocados, one serving is ½ cup. One serving of vegetables is 1 cup of most vegetables, 3 cups of tossed greens, or ½ cup of dense vegetables like beans, corn, peas, or mashed potatoes. Restaurant portions of salads, fruits, or cooked vegetables may be larger than typical single portions, but again, unless you are nearing your goal weight or don't have as much weight to lose, you probably won't have to worry about what counts as a serving right now. Eat all the fruits and vegetables you want, but eat at least five servings a day!

# Preparing Your Fruits and Vegetables

Prepare your fruits and vegetables without added fat or sugar. Fresh, raw vegetables taste great plain, but for variety you can bake, boil, broil, grill, microwave, or steam them. Try combining spices and herbs with your fruits and vegetables, or season them with no-calorie condiments. Caraway, cardamom, coriander, dill, basil, thyme, and marjoram blend well with many vegetables. For an Italian taste, try oregano; for an Indian flavor, try turmeric or curry; for a Mexican feel, add chili powder or cumin. Cinnamon, ginger, cloves, and nutmeg blend well with many fruits. Vinegar, lemon juice, zero-calorie salad dressings, or butter flavorings can also add zest to vegetables and salads. The calorie guideline for dressings and condiments is 15 calories or less per tablespoon. If desired, you can sweeten fruits and salads with Splenda or other artificial sweeteners.

For a special splurge, try an exotic fruit you haven't tried before, such as mango, passion fruit, persimmon, pomegranate, or star fruit. For vegetables, how about artichokes, bok choy, Brussels sprouts, kohlrabi, or Swiss chard? Try an easy veggie dip: Slice some low-calorie vegetables—bell peppers (red are the tastiest), broccoli, carrots, cauliflower, celery, cherry tomatoes, cucumber, or radishes—and dip in 1 tablespoon of fat-free creamy ranch dressing or another dressing of your choice.

If you feel adventurous, try combining fruits and vegetables in salads and cooked dishes. Instead of traditional iceberg lettuce mix, try mixing several different types of salad greens and vegetables. How about bibb lettuce, romaine lettuce, arugula, or radicchio? Add cabbage, broccoli, carrots, mushrooms, tomatoes, chickpeas, radishes, peppers, or any other fresh vegetables. Fruits also go well in salads. Throw in some diced apples, sliced grapes, or raspberries. Several cooked vegetables also combine well together—acorn squash with green peas, carrots and celery, okra and tomatoes, onions and peas, and tomatoes and zucchini.

## Comparison with Other Programs That Use Meal Replacements, Fruits, and Vegetables

In the last chapter, we compared the Simple Diet to other diets that do not use meal replacements to show you why a meal replacement–based diet like the Simple Diet is so effective. In this chapter, we'll compare the Simple Diet to other commercial weight management programs that use meal replacements, fruits, and vegetables.

Compare the weight loss of participants in Jenny Craig,[31] Medifast,[32] and Nutrisystem[33] to our recent report for the Simple Diet.[34] The figure below compares the weight losses for the four programs at three and six months.

Participants using the Simple Diet consisting of five meal replacements (three shakes and two entrées) plus a minimum of five servings of fruits and vegetables lost substantially more weight than participants in the Jenny Craig, Medifast, or Nutrisystem programs. All four groups use prepackaged entrées plus

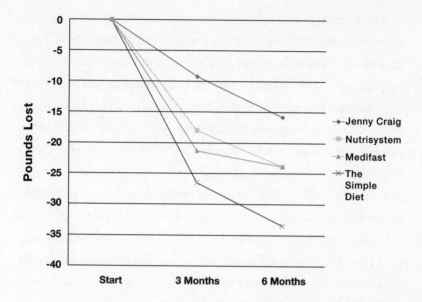

fruits and vegetables, but Jenny Craig and Nutrisystem do not use shakes. Weight losses at three months were: on Jenny Craig, 9.2 pounds; on Nutrisystem, 18 pounds, on Medifast, 21.3 pounds; and on the Simple Diet, 26.5 pounds. Weight losses at six months were: on Jenny Craig, 15.8 pounds; on Nutrisystem, 23.8 pounds; on Medifast, 23.8 pounds; and on the Simple Diet, 33.4 pounds.

I myself used Nutrisystem products for two months. My granddaughter, while living with us for the summer, was enrolled in the Jenny Craig program for three months. Thus I had the opportunity to analyze the nutrition profile of the diet programs to determine how they differ. Using the specific guidance from these two programs—Jenny Craig and Nutrisystem—and those in this book for the Simple Diet, I developed a seven-day menu following the specific instructions from each of the systems and calculated the protein, fat, and calorie contents of each diet for comparison.

Nutrisystem recommends a very healthy diet that is generous in protein and has eight servings of fruits and vegetables. They do not use shakes, but instead recommend Nutrisystem cereal, muffins, or rolls for breakfast and two meal replacements. Following the specific plans outlined, a person would consume about 1,525 calories per day on Nutrisystem, with a food volume of 23 calories per ounce. The dinner entrées that I tried were excellent. Nutrisystem recommends a wide variety of foods that are not portion-controlled. The inclusion of almonds brings in health-promoting monounsaturated fats, but at a high caloric price (90 calories), and the availability of cakes, cookies, and snacks provided temptations that I would rather not have in my kitchen. In short, Nutrisystem provides more options than the Simple Diet, but is likely to yield less weight loss than use of meal replacements, fruits, and vegetables without a number of other options.

Jenny Craig also recommends a very healthy diet using prepackaged entrées, fruits, and vegetables, but does not include shakes. It is more flexible than the other two programs and gives guidelines for use of dairy products and "regular foods." With greater flexibility, weight losses with Jenny Craig appear to be only half of what participants typically lose on the Simple Diet. Jenny Craig does not recommend shakes and uses entrée items for breakfast (cereal, eggs, or pancakes), lunch, and dinner. The program recommends a minimum of four fruits and vegetables in their sample menus. The protein content of the diet is good, and the diet appears to be nutritionally well balanced. Using the minimum food intake recommended with no "regular food" or other choices, the lowest calorie level of the Jenny Craig plan averages 1,453 calories per day, with a volume of 22 calories per ounce. Jenny Craig also offers a variety of foods that are not portion-controlled and includes 23 dessert and snack food choices.

In contrast, the Simple Diet provides about 1,153 calories per day, with a volume of 13 calories per ounce. Thus, the Simple Diet provides much more volume of food for the calories. The only non-portion-controlled foods recommended by the Simple Diet are fruits, vegetables, and condiments with no more than 15 calories per tablespoon. Thus, it appears to me that the use of shakes and the high volume of the recommended foods coupled with the only one snack item (a bar) contributes importantly to the effectiveness of the Simple Diet.

A chart of the approximate nutrition profiles and costs of the three programs is included in the appendix (5.3, Approximate Daily Calorie, Volume, and Nutrition Values for Three Diets).

## Getting in Your Daily Five Fruits and Vegetables

Because of their low energy density and high water content, fruits and vegetables give you a lot of volume and help fill you up without giving you a lot of calories. They are uniquely effective for weight loss and long-term health and weight management because of their low energy density. In fact, the National Weight Control Registry—a real-world database that tallies the behaviors of thousands of people who have lost weight and kept it off—and other careful research show that eating lots of fruits and vegetables is one of the top strategies for long-term weight-loss success.

An added bonus is the terrifically positive example you set for other family members and friends. If you are eating more fruits and vegetables, by virtue of observing you, and also simply because these good foods are consistently stocked in your home, your loved ones may be inspired to eat more fruits and vegetables, too.

Doing some prepping means fresh fruits and vegetables will be handy when you want them. Wash and chop vegetables ahead of time so they are ready to grab. Consider them as great snack choices as well as accompaniment to your entrée at meals. Try blending a variety of fruits into a healthy delicious smoothie, or adding an assortment of vegetables to an entrée meal replacement to create a new dish.

Here are a few of my favorite smoothie recipes. Just add all the ingredients to a blender and blend!

## Chocolate-Strawberry Smoothie

12 oz. cold water

1 Vanilla Pleasure (Revival Soy) shake mix

1 teaspoon dark chocolate cocoa

1 packet sweetener (optional)

4 large strawberries

4 ice cubes

This recipe counts as one shake, one fruit.

## Root Beer–Strawberry Smoothie

6 oz. diet root beer

6 oz. water

1 French Vanilla (Slim-Fast) shake mix

1 packet sweetener (optional)

1 cup frozen strawberries (unsweetened)

4 ice cubes

This recipe counts as one shake, one fruit.

# Strawberry-Banana Smoothie

6 oz. cold water

1 Vanilla (Slim-Rite) shake mix

1 packet sweetener (optional)

½ banana, sliced

1 cup frozen strawberries (unsweetened)

This recipe counts as one shake, two fruits.

# Mixed Berry Fizz

12 oz. Fresca (diet grapefruit soda)

1 Vanilla (GNC) shake mix

1 packet sweetener (optional)

1 cup frozen mixed berries (unsweetened)

This recipe counts as one shake, one fruit.

Hazel, a woman I'll talk more about in the next chapter, got a jump-start on her weight loss by averaging more than seven servings of fruits and vegetables daily in her first week. Her Weekly Summary Sheet is shown below. This thirty-year-old graphic artist jumped into the program enthusiastically and was rewarded with a 7-pound weight loss her first week. Over the first three months in the program, Hazel lost 35 pounds by eating only recommended foods, including seven to nine servings of fruits and vegetables daily. She increased her activity level from that of a desk-bound person to one who burned 3,500 to 4,500 calories during most weeks. She found bars to be convenient when she was focused on projects at work but, with our coaching, found she could get by on less than two bars per day by having fruits or veggies to snack on.

While the basic minimum for the Simple Diet is five servings of fruits and vegetables a day, you are absolutely *not* limited to just five. Look at Hazel's weekly summary sheet. She used seven to nine servings of fruits and vegetables daily and lost an average of 2.7 pounds per week. She told me she liked to add fruit to her shakes and vegetables to her entrées. She said not only was this a great tactic to feel fuller and add variety to her menu, it allowed her to be creative in the kitchen—something she always enjoyed and didn't want to give up when she started the program.

We have found that most people who are successful on the Simple Diet use five to seven meal replacements daily and six to eight servings of fruits and vegetables daily. Many consumed an average of one nutrition bar daily. Following are a few sample menus, showing how you can incorporate shakes, entrées, fruits, and vegetables. Appendix 5.4, The Simple Diet Seven-Day Sample Menus, gives a fuller guide. With choices of dozens of different shakes, hundreds of entrées, and the whole array of fruits and vegetables, you can have a different menu each day for months.

# HAZEL'S WEEKLY SUMMARY SHEET

**BEGINNING DATE: AUG. 8**
**BEGINNING WEIGHT: 207 POUNDS**

| WEEK | SHAKES | ENTRÉES | FRUITS/VEGETABLES | BARS | ON THE DIET* | CONSUMED SEFV** | PHYSICAL ACTIVITY | WEIGHT |
|---|---|---|---|---|---|---|---|---|
| 1 | 25 | 15 | 50 | 8 | 7 | 7 | 2270 | 200 |
| 2 | 21 | 14 | 47 | 12 | 7 | 6 | 3260 | 195.5 |
| 3 | 23 | 15 | 48 | 8 | 7 | 7 | 4579 | 193.5 |
| 4 | 22 | 16 | 50 | 12 | 7 | 6 | 3606 | 190.5 |
| 5 | 23 | 16 | 54 | 16 | 7 | 7 | 4847 | 190.5 |
| 6 | 26 | 16 | 51 | 9 | 7 | 7 | 4385 | 185.5 |
| 7 | 29 | 17 | 56 | 10 | 7 | 7 | 4428 | 184 |
| 8 | 20 | 11 | 31 | 11 | 7 | 4 | 8067 | 182.5 |
| 9 | 27 | 16 | 60 | 15 | 7 | 7 | 4403 | 180 |
| 10 | 26 | 17 | 54 | 11 | 7 | 7 | 4161 | 177.5 |
| 11 | 27 | 15 | 54 | 17 | 7 | 7 | 4009 | 177 |
| 12 | 26 | 14 | 55 | 15 | 7 | 7 | 3571 | 175.5 |
| 13 | 29 | 14 | 63 | 14 | 7 | 7 | 3291 | 172 |

*Consumed only meal replacements, bars, fruits, and vegetables and no other caloric items
**Consumed at least three shakes, two entrées, and five fruits and vegetables (SEFV)

| MEAL | DAY 1 | DAY 2 | DAY 3 |
|---|---|---|---|
| **Breakfast** | Milk Chocolate shake (Special K), 1 whole orange | Rich Chocolate shake (GNC) blended with ½ banana | Vanilla Pleasure shake (Revival Soy) blended with 1 cup frozen mixed berries |
| **Snack** | Cappuccino Delight shake (Slim-Fast), 1 peach | Chocolate Daydream shake (Revival Soy) blended with 1 cup strawberries | Vanilla shake (Slim-Rite) blended with 1 cup blueberries |
| **Lunch** | Ravioli Florentine (Smart Ones) with 2 cups cooked spinach, 1 whole pear | Beef Tips Portobello (Healthy Choice) over baked potato, veggie dip*, 1 whole apple or pear | Chicken Mediterranean (Lean Cuisine) with 1 cup cooked carrots, ½ banana |
| **Snack** | Vanilla Pleasure shake (Revival Soy) blended with 1 cup strawberries | French Vanilla shake (GNC) blended in 12 oz. diet root beer | Rich Chocolate Royale shake (Slim-Fast) blended with 1 cup kiwi |
| **Dinner** | Chicken Santa Fe (Smart Ones), veggie dip*, 1 cup mixed berries | Lasagna with Meat Sauce (Michelina's), 1 cup broccoli, 1 whole peach | Sweet and Sour Chicken (Lean Cuisine), Asian stir-fry vegetables, 1 cup fruit salad |
| **Snack** | French Vanilla shake (Slim-Fast) | Vanilla Bean shake (GNC) blended with frozen mixed fruit | Vanilla shake (Slim-Rite) blended with diet soda and blackberries |
| **Total** | 4 shakes, 2 entrées, 7 fruits and vegetables | 4 shakes, 2 entrées 7 fruits and vegetables | 4 shakes, 2 entrées 8 fruits and vegetables |

* Veggie dip: Select three to five vegetables (bell peppers, broccoli, baby carrots, cauliflower, celery, cherry tomatoes, cucumbers, or radishes); add 1 tbsp. fat-free dressing of your choice. Dip and enjoy.

Even though you now know what you'll be eating on the Simple Diet, eating is only part of the First Phase. When you start increasing your physical activity levels as discussed in the next chapter, you'll be surprised how good you'll feel, not to mention helping those pounds drop off. Chapter 7 will tell you how to keep records, keeping you on the diet and highlighting problem areas, and chapter 8 will give you ideas for gathering support and enlisting your doctor's help. (Remember, you *need* to talk to your doctor before starting the Simple Diet.)

When you've finished reading about the Six Keys, you'll be ready to start your intensive weight loss. The remaining chapters of the book will give suggestions for meeting challenges; guidance on transitioning to the Second Phase, health and weight management; and finally, advice on the Simple Lifetime Diet. Losing weight with the Simple Diet will improve your health and help you enjoy life more.

"I can take charge of my life, and I can use meal replacements, fruits, and vegetables to eat a healthy and weight-maintaining diet."

# 6

# Physical Activity: Step Right This Way

Hazel, a thirty-year-old graphic artist, was five feet five inches tall and weighed 207 pounds. She came to us because she wanted to get back to her pre-college weight. She enthusiastically embraced the physical activity recommendations as she started the program. Initially she focused on walking and soon was logging up to thirty-five miles of walking weekly. To become fit, she joined a gym, where she worked out three days a week doing weight training and aerobic exercise on an elliptical machine. Because of her high levels of physical activity, we encouraged her to use more meal replacements, and some weeks she used up to a total of fifty-two per week. She also consumed up to three bars per day. Over twenty-five weeks, Hazel lost 53 pounds and was happy with a weight of 154 pounds for her large frame.

Increasing your current level of physical activity is *essential* for weight loss and *vital* for long-term weight management. Let's do some arithmetic: To lose two pounds per week, you need to consume 1,000 calories less than your body uses each day. If you are an average 220-pound woman, you burn about 150 calories for each mile you walk, so you can lose two pounds per week by walking about seven miles per day. That's quite a distance! And for most of my patients, that represents a time commitment of two hours and twenty minutes per day! Alternatively, you can lose those two pounds per week if you walk the recommended two miles per day and reduce your calorie intake from about 2,500 calories per day to 1,800 calories per day—an easy task if you follow the Simple Diet. In fact, most individuals in this weight range following the Simple Diet have an even lower caloric intake and lose 2.5 to 3 pounds per week.

I have family members who are very busy—mothers with two or three at-home children—who are on the run all the time (much of it behind the wheel of a car). They ask me, "How can I find the time to be more active?" In our multitasking society, it is a challenge to carve out the time for physical activity. But there are easy ways to work it in and it is essential for weight-loss success.

Yes, some people can lose weight simply by reducing calorie intake, without increasing the level of physical activity, but this is not the case for most people. And even if you are among the 5 percent of people who can lose weight without exercise, physical activity has so many other health benefits, it becomes its own reward. You'll look better, feel better, and have more energy. Exercise also can have a positive effect on numerous health conditions. To increase your probability of being highly successful in this program, we encourage you to plan to increase your physical activity steadily and as quickly as you can.

Also, you do not want to lose 50 pounds this year and find them again next year! We have all had friends who have done that, or have done that ourselves. You are entering a serious weight management training program, with the goal of getting to a health-promoting weight and successfully managing it long-term. Exercise is a vital part of these efforts.

When you exercise, too, you get a lift—your body releases the feel-good endorphin hormones *and* you feel accomplished and successful while you are moving. The positive mood-elevating effects of exercise can give you a boost and make it easier for you to stay on the diet. Research indicates that physical activity serves to attract and hold together other health and weight management behaviors.

In this program, you are also developing habits that will help you manage your health-promoting weight indefinitely. When you move to the Second Phase of the Simple Diet, the health and weight management phase, you'll be able to enjoy a less intense eating plan, using fewer meal replacements and incorporating other foods into your diet. Your newly developed physical activity level will enable you to enjoy these foods while maintaining your weight loss.

## How Much Exercise Does the Trick?

The more exercise, the better. Not surprisingly, people who do more physical activity lose more weight. Studies show that individuals who burned more than 3,000 calories per week lost twice as much weight as those who burned less than 1,000 calories per week in physical activity. We recommend that you burn at least 2,000 calories per week in physical activity.

So how do you burn 2,000 calories in a week? A general guideline, supported by extensive research, is to add the equivalent of walking two miles per day or more, six days per week, to your current activity, whatever that may be. Of course, you can mix and match different forms of physical activity: walking, exercise bicycle, elliptical machine, swimming, aerobics classes at the gym, or water aerobics. In chapter 3, we stressed adding variety in your dietary choices. Variety is also important in your exercise habits, since this makes the activities more fun and strengthens different muscle groups.

Rome wasn't built in a day, and you did not become less physically fit in a day. Set realistic short- and long-term goals for yourself. Maybe you can start out by walking an extra ten minutes twice a day for the first week. Gradually increase this amount, building up to thirty to forty-five minutes of walking six days a week. As illustrated below, a 250-pound person would burn approximately 2,000 calories per week by increasing their walking by about twelve miles per week.

| CURRENT WEIGHT | CALORIES PER MILE | MILES WALKING PER WEEK THAT BURN 2,000 CALORIES PER WEEK* |
|---|---|---|
| 150 pounds | 100 | 20 miles per week |
| 200 pounds | 135 | 15 miles per week |
| 250 pounds | 170 | 12 miles per week |
| 300 pounds | 200 | 10 miles per week |

*Ten minutes of aerobic activity is roughly equivalent to one mile of walking.

I'm occasionally asked, "Do I need to train for a marathon?" No. For many, it's easier to find several smaller pockets of time each day for exercise than to make room for a longer session. And, actually, several short bouts of exercise appear to be more effective than one long bout of exercise. One research study showed that women who routinely got in four ten-minute walks five days per week lost more weight than women who did a single forty-minute session of exercise daily five days per week. Furthermore, the short-burst exercisers showed more diligence; they exercised on 25 percent more days and lost 40 percent more weight.

# What Are the Best Forms of Physical Activity?

While your primary goal is to achieve a health-promoting weight, your objective should also be becoming more physically fit. Physical fitness includes improving cardiovascular fitness, muscle strength, and flexibility. Cardiovascular fitness and health benefits can be achieved by walking, cycling, or using an elliptical machine, or by some other vigorous form of aerobic exercise. So optimal fitness would be achieved by:

- walking coupled with aerobic exercises (cardiovascular fitness);
- weight training (muscle strength); and
- stretching (flexibility).

## ▶ Walking

Most people do some walking in their daily life. We recommend that you increase your walking by small increments to achieve your goals. For most of my patients, increasing their walking is the first step to increasing their fitness. Individuals with arthritis or other limitations in walking abilities can use other strategies as outlined later. The goal is to increase your physical activity to burn 2,000 calories more than you currently burn.

How much do you have to walk to burn an extra 2,000 calories a week? Well, it will vary from person to person, but here are some general guidelines:

First, you need to figure out how much you are currently walking as you go about your day-to-day life. I strongly recommend purchasing a pedometer. A list of recommended pedometers is included in the appendix (6.1, Pedometer Guide). Put the pedometer on your waistband and go about your day. At night, look at your pedometer and see how many steps you've walked. For example, during my average day at home, I take about a thousand steps. I look at this minimum as my basic "couch potato" day. Your goal is to increase your activity to burn an extra 2,000 calories a week. The chart on page 96 shows you approximately how many miles you need to walk to burn those calories.

Next, you need to figure out how many steps you take in a mile. This varies depending on the length of your strides. To be most accurate, you can find a track or a stretch of road that is equal to a mile, walk it, and see how many steps your pedometer records. However, you could also estimate; the average is two thousand steps per mile.

So if you weigh 200 pounds, you need to increase your walking by thirty thousand steps per week (15 miles x 2,000 steps), or five thousand steps per day, six days a week (30,000 steps ÷ 6 days). Remember, that's five thousand steps *more* than what you do on your average "couch potato" day.

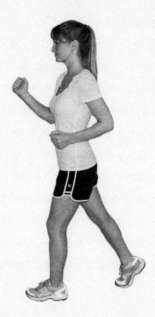

This may seem like a lot, but you can increase your steps gradually and find simple ways to add steps: take the stairs instead of the elevator, take a ten-minute walk at lunch; walk with your family after dinner.

Your pedometer can serve as a coach, encouraging you to meet your daily goals. People who use pedometers say that getting in their daily steps is more like fun than dutiful exercise, a game they're constantly playing. Find ways to increase your walking. Select the most distant parking space rather than circling the parking lot several times to park near the store or office. Return the shopping cart to the front of the store rather than leaving it in the middle of the parking lot. Walk around during TV commercials or when on boring conference calls. Every little bit counts.

Any effort that burns calories improves cardiovascular health and wellness. Walking is one of the healthiest activities you can do and is associated with fewer injuries and downtime than more vigorous exercise such as running. Try a race-walking style with elbows bent to slightly less than 90 degrees and pumping your fists in front of you as you walk (see figure on previous page).

Practicing this form of walking may help you subtly increase your pace over time. Many people, even a seventy-five-year-old guy like me, can walk a mile in less than fifteen minutes, or more than four miles per hour. Both walking and using an exercise bicycle in a low-intensity effort improve cardiovascular fitness. Amanda (chapter 8) and Denise (chapter 4) were walkers who preferred to burn calories mainly by walking at a brisk pace, while Hazel (chapters 5 and 6) preferred to go to the gym three times a week for weight training to improve strength and muscle tone.

## ▶ Aerobic Exercise

While walking is a very effective way to improve cardiovascular fitness, down the road you may want to add some sort of more intense aerobic exercise to improve endurance. Aerobic exercises are exercises that use large muscle groups, causing the heart and lungs to work harder than they do at rest. Leisurely walking burns calories and improves your fitness but does not cause your heart rate or breathing to increase very much. If you pedal your exercise bicycle at a low resistance and a moderate rate (maybe while reading a book), you are burning calories, but you are not enhancing your aerobic fitness. If your bicycle has a heart monitor, you'll see that your pulse rate probably stays under 100 beats per minute. To become more aerobically fit, however, you'll have to push the envelope by increasing the resistance and pedaling faster. With this increased intensity, your heart rate will increase to over 100 beats per minute and you will start breathing harder. Aerobic fitness is documented to increase cognition and to reduce cardiovascular disease.

As a general goal, you would like for your heart rate to go to about 65 to 85 percent of your maximum heart rate (calculated as 220 minus your age). So if you are forty years old, your maximum heart rate is 180 beats per minute (220 - 40) and your target heart rate would be from 117 beats per minute (0.65 x 180) up to 153 beats per minute (0.85 x 180). As a general rule, I recommend you try to keep your heart rate around 75 percent of your maximum (see the table below). Doing about ten minutes at this level of intensity is approximately equivalent to walking one mile and enhances your aerobic fitness. You can also do this on a treadmill, on an elliptical machine, in a Spinning or Pilates class, or with water aerobics.

| AGE | TARGET HEART RATE (65–85% MAXIMUM) BEATS PER MINUTE | RECOMMENDED LEVEL BEATS PER MINUTE |
|---|---|---|
| 20 | 130–170 | 150 |
| 30 | 124–162 | 143 |
| 40 | 117–153 | 135 |
| 50 | 111–145 | 128 |
| 60 | 104–136 | 120 |
| 70 | 98–128 | 113 |

*Paul was a thirty-six-year-old man who operated a dance studio and had been an active instructor until he injured his back in an auto accident. With the lack of physical activity, he had gained weight and was carrying almost 250 pounds—much too much for his height of five feet eleven inches. He was frustrated and depressed because, at this weight, he could not effectively provide dance instructions. His back was improving with physical therapy, and he was determined to get back to his active dancing weight. When he first came to me, he weighed in at 242 pounds and began using three shakes, two entrées, and at least seven servings of fruits and vegetables daily.*

*Over the first four weeks, Paul lost 26 pounds and increased his physical activity from 1,000 to 3,000 calories per week by walking twenty minutes twice a day, six days a week. He was very disciplined and did not eat any food that was not on the Simple Diet. The initial weight loss of more than 6 pounds per week had restored his confidence, and his depression lifted noticeably at his weekly visits. Over the next twelve weeks, he lost another 34 pounds, getting down to a weight of 184 pounds. He was so excited that he could resume teaching his classes several evenings weekly.*

*Over the next six months, Paul continued to use several shakes or entrées and consumed six to eight servings of fruits and vegetables daily. With this regimen, he achieved his pre-injury weight of 175 pounds and is maintaining that weight. He is back to his energetic and enthusiastic self and off all pain and antidepressant medications.*

## ▶ Weight Training

Weight training is another health-promoting activity and has the added benefit of toning up trouble spots. Do you have "wings" under your upper arms that flap when you clap? These are very flabby triceps muscles and skin with lots of excessive fat accumulation. Including weight training in your physical activity plan will help tone up these wings, as well as strengthen other muscle groups throughout the body.

I have developed a pattern of weight training that has been reviewed and endorsed by trainers at three different gyms I have visited. I use very common exercises that you are probably already familiar with, but if you are not, there are several books or videos you can use. Some of these are listed in the appendix (6.2, Recommended Exercise Guides). For maximum muscle strengthening, exercises should be done slowly and not with a swinging motion. Pause for one or two seconds at the completion of each weight movement and again in the resting position.

Begin with the first five weight training exercises, then add the other seven exercises as quickly as you can without more than mild aching of your muscle after the training set.

**Seated biceps curls:** Sitting on an armless chair or bench, start with the dumbbells at your sides. With your palms facing forward, curl both arms, slowly raising the weights to your shoulders. Lower the dumbbells to the starting position. Keep your torso still. Avoid swinging the weights up.

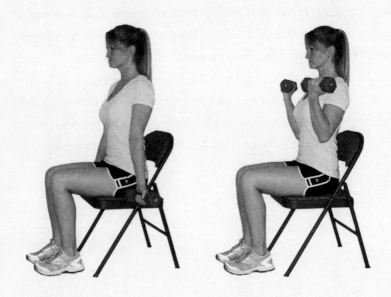

## Seated triceps curls:

Seated with the dumbbell in your left hand, raise the weight all the way behind your head with the arm curled and the weight beside your left ear; push the left elbow back with the right hand. Slowly uncurl the arm to the straightened position. Slowly return the weight to the starting position. Avoid swinging the weight. Repeat the same exercise with the dumbbell in your right hand.

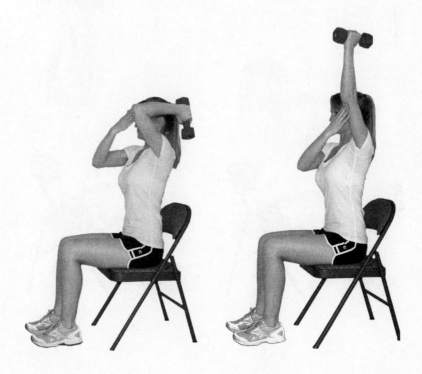

**Seated dumbbell press:** Seated with both arms flexed, holding the dumbbells even with your chin and your palms facing your chin, raise the weights straight upward slowly to fully extend the arms. Pause, and then slowly lower the dumbbells to the starting position. Pause and repeat.

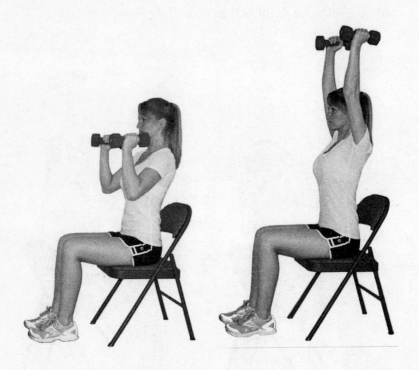

**Seated dumbbell fly:** Seated with the dumb-bells in each hand with your arms extended at shoulder level and palms facing forward, slowly bring the weights together in front of your face, keeping your arms extended forward. Pause and slowly return to starting position.

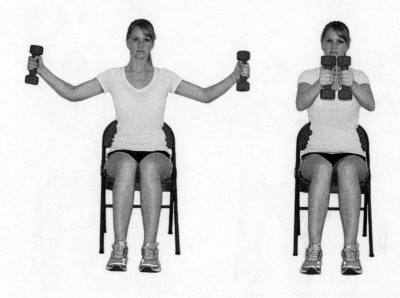

**Seated dumbbell butterfly:** Seated with the dumbbells in each hand extended at shoulder level with palms facing up, slowly raise the weights to meet directly above your head. Return slowly to the starting position, pause, and repeat.

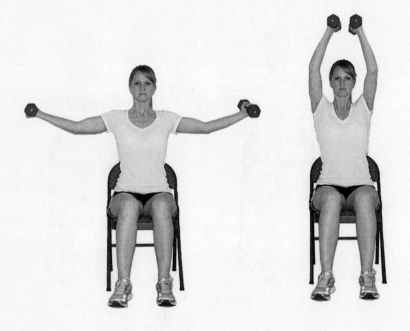

## Straight leg raise: Seated with both feet on the floor, slowly extend the left leg as far forward as possible. Pause, then slowly return to the starting position. Pause and repeat. Repeat with the right leg. This also can be done after muscles are more developed with weights around each ankle.

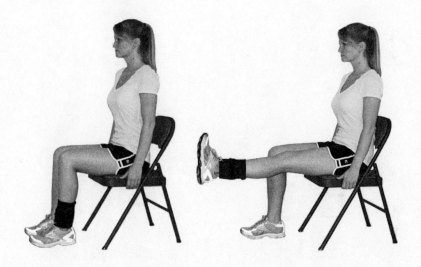

**Angled calf raise:** Standing with both dumbbells at your sides about six inches lateral to the hips and with toes pointed outward at a 30-degree angle, slowly stand on tiptoes and pause. Return slowly to starting position, pause, and repeat.

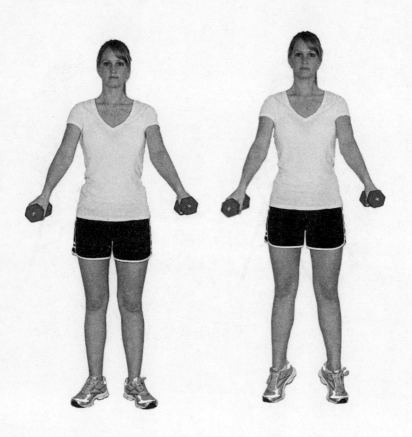

**Prone leg flexion:** Lying comfortably on your stomach on a mat, slowly bend your left leg as far as possible while keeping your foot flexed. Pause and return to starting position. Repeat with the right leg. Can be done with or without ankle weights.

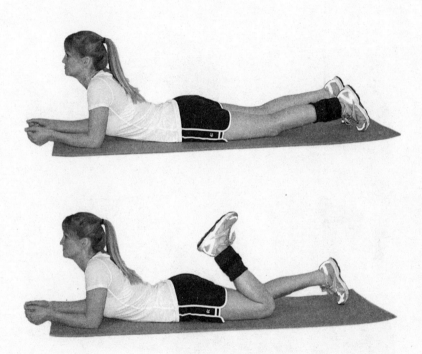

**Supine dumbbell fly:** Lying on your back with weights in both hands and arms extended at shoulder level, slowly raise both arms off the floor to meet extended directly above your chest. Pause and return slowly to the starting position to rest hands and weights on the floor. Repeat slowly.

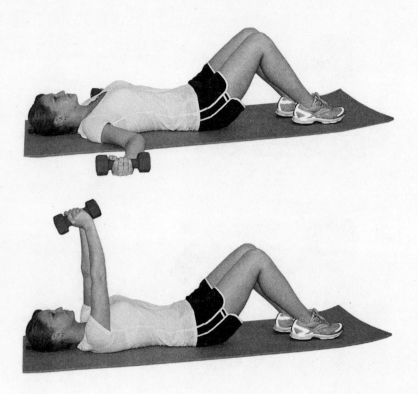

**Supine dumbbell press:** Lying on your back with weights in each hand and lower arms bent so that your hands are slightly above your chest, raise arms straight above you to have the weights meet with your arms extended. Pause and return slowly to the starting position.

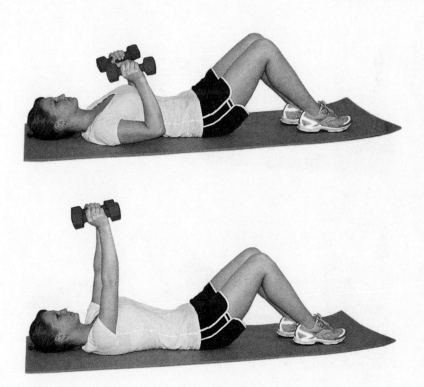

## Supine dumbbells over head: Lying on your back holding weights beside your hips with palms facing hips, slowly raise the weights and continue the movement until the weights come together touching the floor above your head. Pause and slowly return to starting position. Pause and slowly repeat exercise.

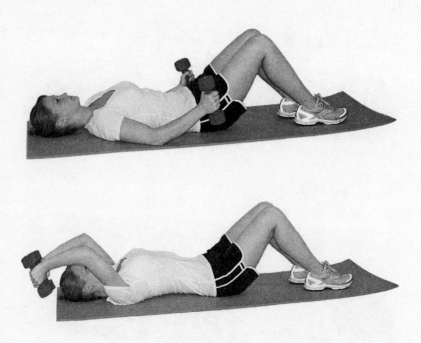

**Abdominal crunches:** Lying on your back with knees bent, feet flat on the floor, and arms to your sides, slowly bend forward, moving your hands with palms down until fingers approach or touch knees. Pause, and then slowly return to starting position. Pause and repeat.

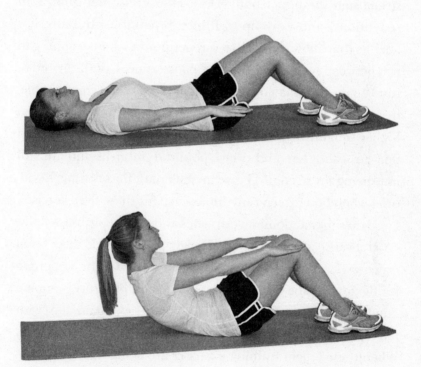

I suggest starting with three- or five-pound weights. Do ten biceps curls without stopping; choose the weight that makes doing the ten reps just a bit of a challenge. When that weight gets too easy, you can increase weight or increase the number of repetitions.

Since you are walking or doing some cardiovascular exercises that work the legs, start with the first five exercises that strengthen the upper body. Do each exercise ten times (ten repetitions) and work up to fifteen repetitions. Initially, use weights that allow you to do ten repetitions without stopping to rest between reps, except for the pause at peak position and at rest. Do movements slowly without jerking. When you feel able, increase to fifteen repetitions. When this gets easy, use the next higher weight; I started out using five-pound dumbbells and now am using ten- and twelve-pound dumbbells and am still improving my strength. I give myself credit for burning 75 calories when I do fifteen repetitions each for these five exercises. I also do thirty abdominal crunches and fifteen push-ups daily.

To advance to a fuller-ranging weight program, add these seven exercises: straight leg raise (no weights), angled calf raise, prone leg flexion, supine dumbbell fly, supine dumbbell press, supine dumbbells over head, and abdominal crunches. Again, start with ten repetitions with comfortable weights and build up to fifteen. When these weight training exercises are going well, add push-ups. You can start with full push-ups or with push-ups from the knees rather than the toes (see figure on next page).

I started with three (!) and now do fifteen to twenty-five, six evenings a week. For counting calories, I count one calorie per weight repetition, crunch, or push-up. When I do my full workout at home, I estimate that I burn about 225 calories. I recommend doing weight training three times a week.

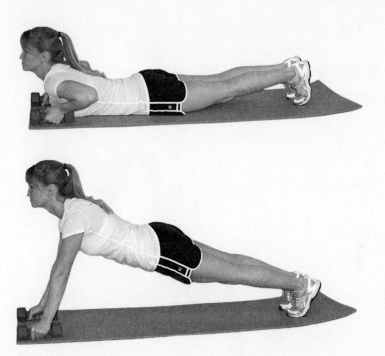

To advance to a more complete weight training program, I suggest joining a gym or enrolling at your local YMCA. This way, a trainer can offer guidance on which machines to use and how to use them safely and most effectively.

## Flexibility

Flexibility is the third component of fitness. Being a slow learner, I only started working on flexibility three years ago. Achieving and maintaining flexibility decreases risks of muscle, joint, and tendon injuries and risk of falls. Hold each stretch position for fifteen seconds by counting to fifteen by thousands (one thousand one, one thousand two, etc.). The eight stretches that I recommend and do are these:

**Dumbbell squat:** Squat as far as possible with dumbbells in each hand extended above your knees.

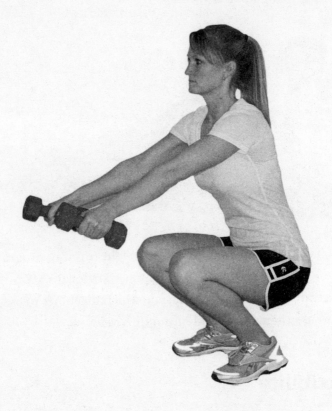

**Alternating lunges:** Squatting with the left knee at a 90-degree angle and the right leg extended behind you, hold dumbbells out about six to nine inches above your knees; repeat with right leg extended forward and left leg behind.

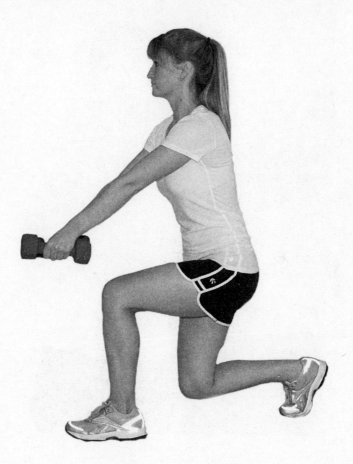

**Pectoral stretches:** With your right hand above your left breast (flag salute position), press your left palm against a doorway. Repeat, stretching opposite chest muscles.

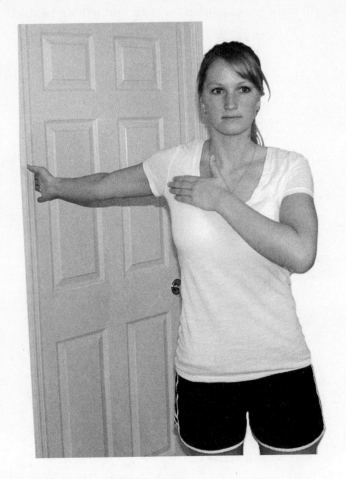

## Deltoid stretches: With your left arm extended across your right shoulder and your right arm flexed around your left elbow, stretch the deltoid. Repeat with your right arm extended.

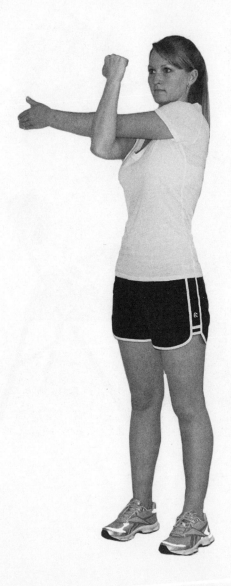

**Triceps stretches:** Raise the left elbow above the left shoulder with the left arm fully flexed. Push the left elbow back slightly with the right hand. Repeat with the right arm.

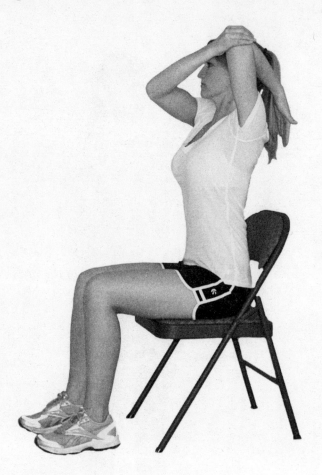

**Toe touch:** Bend forward with your knees straight and stretch to touch your toes with your fingertips. You may not be able to reach your toes initially, but keep pushing!

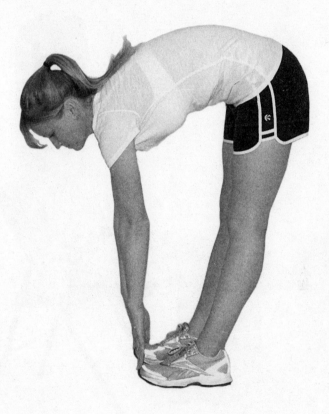

**Straight-leg stretches:** Sitting in a chair, stretch the left leg forward in front of you as far as possible. Repeat with the right leg.

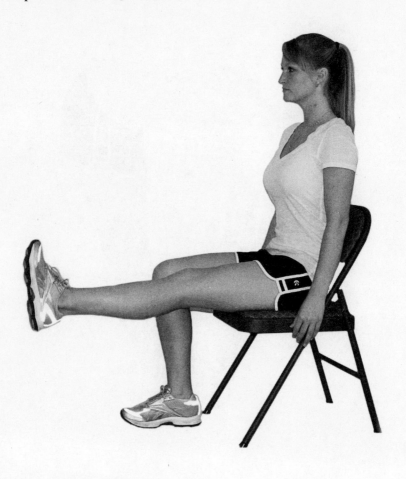

## Prone-leg stretches: Lying on your stomach, flex the left leg as far forward as possible, holding the leg forward with the left hand pulling on the foot. Repeat with right leg.

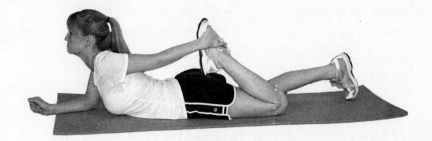

Stretching takes only a few minutes, and I recommend you do these after your exercises.

All three types of fitness training are important. Under ideal circumstances, I would recommend this balance: ten to twenty minutes of aerobic training with your heart rate in the target range three times weekly, about forty-five minutes of weight training three times weekly, race-style walking on three days per week, and stretching six days per week. Continue doing push-ups six days per week.

## If Your Mobility Is Limited

I often have patients who have limitations in walking. One fifty-six-year-old woman, at 330 pounds, was disabled with arthritis of both knees and used a motorized wheelchair to get around. In our discussion, she indicated that she could do limited walking around the kitchen and to the bathroom from her bed. We agreed that she could try walking from the kitchen to the bedroom and back after each meal. She was able to do this, and as she lost weight she increased her walking at home. After several weeks she mentioned that her granddaughter loved to shop and that the wheelchair limited her mobility in shops at the mall. We decided that she could leave the wheelchair outside the shop and walk around inside. After several more weeks, she announced that her granddaughter was dropping her off at the entrance to the mall and she was walking around, resting periodically at the benches in the corridors. After losing 50 pounds, she was walking from end to end in the mall and had become a shopaholic.

Some individuals have substantial limitations and cannot walk at all. I recently worked with a forty-five-year-old man who had bilateral above-knee amputations after an accident at work. He does physical therapy and pool work with a therapist and burns over 5,000 calories per week! Another sixty-one-year-old woman had a motorized wheelchair because of severe arthritis. She started with upper body exercises and limited water aerobics, and after losing 80 pounds, she has turned in her handicapped sticker and walks everywhere. Recently, I counseled a sixty-seven-year-old man with severe arthritis of the knees to explore water aerobics and begin some of the dumbbell weight-lifting exercises outlined above. We are able to tailor some sort of physical activity to encourage all of our patients to increase their activity. Where there's a will, there's a way!

## Adding Up Your Calories

Let's review the calculation of your daily calorie burn. If you weigh about 200 pounds, you burn about 135 calories per mile of walking. If you walk two miles, that's 270 calories. If you spend ten minutes on an exercise bicycle at a moderate speed and intensity, that would be about one mile's worth, or 135 calories. At the gym, if you do fifteen repetitions with weights that have you feeling it with the last few reps, that's approximately 15 calories per exercise, 150 calories if you do ten exercises. When you do stretching for fifteen seconds, you can count that as 5 calories per stretch maneuver, or 40 calories for eight stretching maneuvers. (Some of the weight and stretching calorie estimations I provide may not be exactly accurate, but I would rather be a little generous here in order to encourage you to do these important training activities.) In total, this level of physical activity adds up to almost 600 calories daily. If you did this six days a week, you'd be burning 3,570 calories—enough for about an additional pound of weight loss weekly!

# Records Keep You Focused

In medicine, we say that if you didn't record it, you didn't do it. Keeping daily records of your physical activity is very important because it keeps you focused on your task and your goals.

When recording your activity, remember to only count activity *above* your baseline "couch potato" rate. For example, when I finish my *active* day, I subtract my one thousand "couch potato" steps from my total and determine how many steps and miles I have taken *above* that minimum. We recommend that you *increase* your walking or other equivalent activity to two miles per day, six days a week. Each evening, record your mileage and calories burned when you record your shake, entrée, fruit, and vegetable intake. (See appendices 3.3 and 3.4 for daily progress and weekly summary charts you can copy.)

Partner with a friend or relative who is interested in your health and fitness. Share with them your daily totals in person, by phone, or over e-mail. You may find that you can empower this individual to improve their own physical fitness. Or maybe you have a friend who is a fitness buff with missionary zeal who would be pleased to hear about your progress. At my YMCA, I can share my progress with my trainer several times weekly, although I only have scheduled time with him biweekly.

*Brenda, the twenty-four-year-old graduate student whose story we shared with you in chapter 3, was a former college athlete excited about enrolling in the program and beginning the Simple Diet. She believed that resuming regular physical activity and the flexibility of the diet would enable her to lose weight quickly, and she was right! Brenda kept good records, but the challenges of resuming school in the fall and her busy academic and social schedule made it difficult for her to avoid foods that were not on the diet. Nevertheless, with our encouragement, she consumed the minimum recommended shakes and entrées on most days and averaged over 2,000 calories a week in physical activity. She lost 36 pounds over eleven weeks and continued to lose weight after transitioning to the health and weight management phase of the program. She felt that keeping records really enhanced her ability to track her activities and monitor her behavior. Her weekly record is on the next page.*

**BEGINNING DATE: AUG. 6**
**BEGINNING WEIGHT: 203.5**

| WEEK | SHAKES | ENTRÉES | FRUITS/VEGETABLES | BARS | ON THE DIET* | CONSUMED SEFV** | PHYSICAL ACTIVITY | WEIGHT |
|---|---|---|---|---|---|---|---|---|
| 1 | 22 | 14 | 36 | 0 | 7 | 7 | 2900 | 195 |
| 2 | 21 | 13 | 35 | 1 | 6 | 6 | 2600 | 190.5 |
| 3 | 21 | 15 | 37 | 1 | 6 | 7 | 2760 | 187 |
| 4 | 24 | 14 | 39 | 1 | 6 | 7 | 2400 | 182.5 |
| 5 | 29 | 14 | 45 | 2 | 6 | 7 | 1920 | 180 |
| 6 | 28 | 14 | 42 | 0 | 6 | 7 | 2070 | 179 |
| 7 | 28 | 14 | 43 | 1 | 6 | 7 | 3195 | 174.5 |
| 8 | 32 | 13 | 45 | 0 | 6 | 6 | 2800 | 173 |
| 9 | 29 | 15 | 45 | 1 | 6 | 7 | 1320 | 171 |
| 10 | 28 | 14 | 43 | 1 | 6 | 7 | 1500 | 168.5 |
| 11 | 28 | 14 | 43 | 1 | 5 | 7 | 1500 | 167.5 |

*Consumed only meal replacements, bars, fruits, and vegetables and no other caloric items
**Consumed at least three shakes, two entrées, and five fruits and vegetables (SEFV)

# Health Benefits of Physical Activity

Jeff, the fifty-three-year-old fireman you met in the last chapter, experienced firsthand the health benefits of physical activity. Jeff was able to discontinue insulin and all medications as he lost weight, began working with a personal trainer, and walked.

The strong recommendation of experts is thirty to forty-five minutes daily of walking or equivalent exercise for sustained weight loss. Our own research indicates that increasing physical activity by 2,000 calories per week (walking two miles per day, six days a week) sustains a very satisfactory rate of weight loss.[35]

In addition to its vital role in weight maintenance, moderate to high levels of physical activity or fitness have broad health benefits, improving longevity and decreasing the risks for many diseases, which we will talk more about in chapter 12. High levels of physical fitness significantly reduce risk for death from heart attacks in women and men. Women with high levels of physical fitness have a 70 percent lower rate of death from coronary heart disease than do women with low levels of fitness. Similarly, men with high levels of physical fitness have a 50 percent lower rate of death from heart disease than do men with low levels of physical fitness.

Dr. JoAnn Manson at Harvard University has done very persuasive research showing that the risk of developing coronary heart disease is closely associated with an individual's level of physical activity. The more active a woman is, the lower her risk for heart attack. Women who have very high levels of physical activity have a 45 percent lower risk of developing heart disease than do women with very low levels of physical activity.

Dr. Manson has further demonstrated that women who never walk have the highest risk for heart attacks. A woman who walks the average rate of 2.5 miles per hour (one mile in twenty-four minutes) has a 14 percent reduction in heart attack risk, while a woman who walks briskly at 3.5 miles per hour (one mile in seventeen minutes) has a 24 percent reduction in risk. Very brisk walking women (4.5 miles per hour or one mile in thirteen to fourteen minutes) have a 42 percent reduction in risk. You can see why we want you to pick up your pace in walking!

## Step This Way

It should now be quite clear that increasing your physical activity is essential for weight loss and vital for long-term health and weight management. Even if you are moderately active, if you are reading this book, it should be clear to you that this level of physical activity has not maintained your weight at a desirable level. To improve your weight, you will need to improve your physical activity and fitness. More physical activity helps with both your weight loss and your overall health.

"I can use the positive effects of exercise in my life to give me even more motivation to exercise at least six days per week."

# Recordkeeping

## 7

Keeping a daily written record of all your successes—eating your five meal replacements and five servings of fruits and vegetables and burning 2,000 or more extra calories with physical activity weekly—makes you much more likely to achieve your weight-loss and -management goals.

My patients have told me that recordkeeping helps them make the right food choices. If you are debating whether or not to eat that chocolate-covered doughnut and know you have to *write down* the fact that you went off the diet plan, you might decide to pass. Likewise, seeing that you didn't walk much yesterday, you're more likely to increase your physical activity level today.

Recordkeeping, including both daily progress and weekly summary charts, can also inspire and motivate you by showing the progress you've made toward meeting your goals. Say, for example, that you started out walking only ten minutes daily at a slow pace, perhaps burning only 60 or 70 extra calories daily.

It's inspiring to see that, after a few weeks, you're now walking up to thirty to forty minutes daily, burning four or five times the amount of calories. You may even start competing with yourself, trying to beat your own daily activity record. That's a win-win situation!

Recordkeeping also helps you view your weight loss realistically. Maybe you're not losing as much weight as you would like to. Well, it's easier to understand why when you can quickly analyze whether you've stayed on the diet; included at least the minimum recommended servings of shakes, entrées, fruits, vegetables, and fluid; and burned the recommended amount of calories weekly. You might forget what you did to help you lose weight, but a written summary won't forget. You can refer back to it for ideas when you face difficult days or challenges.

# Why Records Help

In our experience, recordkeeping is a critical component of the Simple Diet.

In your golfing or bowling game, you can't improve if you don't know your score. It's the same with losing weight: Keeping records is a way of keeping track of where you are so you know how you're doing and where you can improve.

Individuals like you and me who need to work on weight management appear to have distinct differences from our slender friends who can eat anything. Some of them, like my trim wife, are fidgeters—always active, always moving their legs, getting up from the dinner table multiple times. They have what Dr. James Levine of the Mayo Clinic calls *non-exercise activity thermogenesis* (or NEAT)—they burn calories without even realizing it through their constant motion. Other slender people have other attributes that allow them to remain slender. I live to eat, am a volume eater, and love desserts, while my wife eats to live, is a nibbler, and often eats only half of a dessert (imagine that!).

We probably can't change these tendencies that have genetic, familial, and environmental components, so we overweight-prone people need to develop other behaviors to achieve and keep a healthy weight. We can change habits, but it takes work and practice. Research psychologists tell us that recordkeeping is one of the most important strategies for developing and maintaining these new behaviors and habits—a process they call *cognitive restructuring*. Raising self-awareness through recordkeeping is an essential first step for behavior change. Practicing positive self-talk will reinforce these new habits. ("I can use my records to learn how health-management activities contribute to my wellness.")

And it works. Studies repeatedly show that people who actually write down their food intake and activity levels are more successful at losing weight and keeping it off. The National Weight Control Registry of people who have kept off an average weight loss of 66 pounds for an average of 5.5 years shows that people who keep the weight off share common behavioral strategies, including keeping frequent written records of body weight and food intake.[36]

Keeping daily progress and weekly summary charts offers many benefits. Many people eat without even realizing what they are eating. The simple act of writing something down makes you more aware of it. As I'll discuss in the next chapter, keeping records builds commitment to the program and provides a form of accountability. Many of us will avoid going off the diet if we know we have to write it down.

Keeping records also helps us recognize potential problem areas and test solutions. We can see trends and patterns more clearly on paper. If you notice your weight loss is slowing and can see a correlation between the slowdown and days you don't always include the minimum recommended servings of shakes and entrées or days that you are off the diet, this should tell you it's time to practice adding volume and variety—eating more shakes, entrées, fruits, and vegetables—and not whatever that other stuff was, most certainly higher-calorie foods. With written records, you'll be able to see at a quick glance how the eating-more strategy helps you stay on the diet and drop more weight.

Keeping records also gives you motivation to continue the diet when you see the positive changes over time. You'll begin to see that you can expect steady weight loss when you regularly eat at least the minimum recommended servings, stay on the diet, and fulfill your commitment to increasing your physical activity. Writing down your positive weight-loss behaviors will spur you to do more of them.

## What You Need to Track

Keeping track of your progress doesn't have to be a big, complicated affair. It's really very simple and should only involve fewer than ten minutes of your time daily.

Appendices 3.3 and 3.4 provide templates of daily progress and weekly summary charts that you can photocopy and use. We also showed you (in chapter 3) the completed charts for Angie, the third-grade teacher who was losing weight before her twentieth wedding anniversary trip to Hawaii.

You can use the charts we provide, create your own charts, use Excel spreadsheets or your smartphone—really, any means you prefer. The important information to keep track of in your daily record includes:

- the number of shakes, entrées, bars, and servings of fruits and vegetables daily;
- whether you stayed on the diet (ate *only* foods/beverages on the Simple Diet);
- whether you included at least the minimum number of servings of shakes (three), entrées (two), fruits and vegetables (five); and
- the number of *additional* calories expended in physical activity daily beyond calories you used to expend before you started the program.

Note: For the Simple Diet, I am not asking you to write down everything you eat or keep track of points, calories, fat, or carbohydrate intake.

At the end of the week, add up your weekly totals for shakes, entrées, fruits, vegetables, and bars; days on the diet; days you included at least the minimum recommended number of servings of shakes, entrées, fruits, and vegetables; and additional calories burned in physical activity. Add your weekly weight to this chart and you have an extremely useful tool to help you track your progress and meet challenges.

The table on the next page shows the weekly summary chart for Denise, the fifty-six-year-old grandmother you met in chapter 4.

**BEGINNING DATE: JAN. 22**
**BEGINNING WEIGHT: 233.5**

| WEEK | SHAKES | ENTRÉES | FRUITS/VEGETABLES | BARS | ON THE DIET* | CONSUMED SEFV** | PHYSICAL ACTIVITY | WEIGHT |
|---|---|---|---|---|---|---|---|---|
| 1 | 21 | 14 | 36 | 0 | 6 | 7 | 575 | 228.5 |
| 2 | 21 | 14 | 35 | 0 | 7 | 6 | 1280 | 223.5 |
| 3 | 19 | 13 | 38 | 0 | 7 | 5 | 1580 | 220 |
| 4 | 21 | 15 | 36 | 0 | 7 | 7 | 1795 | 217.5 |
| 5 | 21 | 14 | 36 | 1 | 7 | 7 | 2360 | 213 |
| 6 | 21 | 14 | 38 | 0 | 7 | 7 | 2150 | 209.5 |
| 7 | 21 | 14 | 35 | 2 | 7 | 7 | 2130 | 207.5 |
| 8 | 20 | 14 | 34 | 0 | 7 | 6 | 1910 | 204 |
| 9 | 21 | 14 | 41 | 0 | 7 | 7 | 2200 | 201 |
| 10 | 21 | 16 | 41 | 0 | 7 | 7 | 2230 | 198.5 |
| 11 | 21 | 14 | 41 | 0 | 7 | 7 | 2485 | 194.5 |
| 12 | 20 | 12 | 41 | 0 | 6 | 6 | 2235 | 192 |
| 13 | 21 | 14 | 36 | 0 | 6 | 7 | 2375 | 190 |

*Consumed only meal replacements, bars, fruits, and vegetables and no other caloric items
**Consumed at least three shakes, two entrées, and five fruits and vegetables

With a beginning weight of 233.5 pounds, Denise diligently followed the program and lost weight steadily throughout her thirteen weeks on the Simple Diet. She lost 10 pounds the first two weeks on the program and continued to lose 2 to 4.5 pounds every week thereafter. Over three months she dropped more than 43 pounds.

As her summary chart shows, Denise stayed on the diet all but three days during her thirteen weeks on the program. She almost always included the minimum number of servings of shakes, entrées, fruits, and vegetables. She kept diligent records, and although she wasn't 100 percent perfect on the diet, no one could argue with her success at losing weight. The last time I saw Denise, she weighed 140 pounds and was still using shakes and entrées daily and enjoying fruits and vegetables like she had never done before.

Numerous studies show that recordkeeping not only helps you lose weight, but also helps you manage your weight long-term. For example, if you weigh in weekly and record your weight, you'll be more successful keeping off the pounds. The key is accountability. If you know that when you overdo it you'll have to face the scale in the morning and write down your weight, you'll be less likely to overdo it!

# How to Keep Records

You don't need to write down every bite as you eat it or jot down every step you take. Just three times a day, fill out your daily progress chart, entering the number of shakes, entrées, and bars used, the servings of fruits and vegetables, and the physical activity calories beyond what you normally expend.

Start after breakfast with your new line for the day and plan for the morning. In the afternoon, complete your morning and lunch information and plan for the evening. I use my midday review to decide on my choices of meal replacements and fruits and vegetables, and to plan my physical activity for the afternoon and evening. If you wait until bedtime to complete your daily chart, you may be tired and may not remember all the details of your day. Besides, at bedtime you can't change your food or exercise behavior for the day! In the evening, add up your total daily physical activity, evaluate your positive behaviors and any suboptimal ones, and make a plan for the next day. Use check boxes to indicate days you stayed on the diet as well as days you consumed at least the minimum servings of shakes, entrées, fruits, and vegetables.

Try to keep your daily program record with you at all times, wherever you go. This helps maintain awareness of your commitment and serves as a reminder of your motivation. If you do forget to take your program record with you, jot down your food and calorie burn information on a slip of paper and enter it in later. Make recordkeeping a habit as routine as brushing your teeth.

As you complete your records for the day, look at things that worked for you and things that didn't work. For example, suppose after a long walk you had two bars (2 ounces and 320 calories) and were still hungry. What works for me after a four-mile walk is to have a double shake with a cup of strawberries (24 ounces of fluid and 245 calories). Or you may try having an entrée such as a Smart Ones Chicken Marsala (8 ounces and 160 calories) instead of the two bars.

Keeping your daily record builds accountability; it is always there, acts as your conscience, and will help you stay on the "write" track—the happy, healthy track of losing weight and keeping it off. At the end of the week, transfer the information from your daily chart to your weekly summary chart, where trends over time become even more evident. Give yourself a high five for your successes and plan for your next week. Looking at your weekly summary chart helps you see the big picture, helps you lay out a plan for the next week, and reinforces the diet-positive actions you've taken in previous weeks.

## How Often to Weigh Yourself

Weighing yourself is an important part of self-monitoring and recording. I recommend that you obtain a reliable scale and weigh yourself in the buff daily before breakfast. I don't write these weights down, but they do give me a general sense of progress and daily fluctuations. Near the end of the week, weigh yourself on two different days, maybe Saturday and Sunday. Because of fluctuations in water weight and contents of the GI tract, an average of two weights is better than relying on a single weight. I average these two values for my end of the week weight and write that value down on my weekly summary chart.

## Learning from Your Records

Daily and weekly records provide valuable information to help you fine-tune your weight-loss strategies. If you are having trouble staying on the diet because you are hungry, for example, you can boost your intake of fruits, vegetables, and meal replacements and/or boost the volume of these foods to help you through this time period. You may also want to jot down if you are having any particular challenges on a given day, such as dealing with a food-focused social event, traveling, or eating out at a restaurant. Having a written record of how you dealt with one challenge will help you conquer future challenges. You can also spot trends in diet compliance and amounts of physical activity relative to weight loss quickly when you compare weekly outcomes on your summary chart.

> *Wayne was a fifty-one-year-old Lexmark executive who had participated in an earlier version of the program that had included only shakes and entrées. He was enthusiastic about the Simple Diet because it included fruits and vegetables, and he had previously struggled with the limitations of a diet of just shakes and entrées. Wayne's oldest daughter had just graduated from college and was soon getting married. Wayne wanted to lose weight before the wedding and looked forward to being a grandfather in the future.*
>
> *Before Wayne started his current weight-loss effort, we discussed using fruits and vegetables to meet his need to have a large volume of food. In addition to his high blood pressure (three medicines), high blood fats (two medicines), and indigestion (one medicine), he now had prediabetes. At five feet eleven inches tall and weighing 320 pounds, Wayne needed to lose over 100 pounds to achieve a health-promoting weight for his large frame.*
>
> *Wayne blocked out six months on his busy calendar to religiously follow the diet and exercise plan. We discussed using a minimum of three shakes, two entrées, and seven*

*servings of fruits and vegetables daily (more if needed), as*
*well as walking at least two miles daily. Because his father*
*had died from complications related to diabetes, Wayne was*
*serious about losing weight and keeping it off.*

*An engineer, Wayne began tabulating his diet and*
*physical activities daily on a spreadsheet. He followed the*
*recommended food choices, staying on the diet, but did not*
*always consume the minimum number of shakes and entrées.*
*He began walking around his facility and logged at least two*
*miles daily, losing 62 pounds in ten weeks. We helped him*
*taper off two blood pressure medicines and one lipid*
*medicine. After twenty-four weeks, he had dropped 111*
*pounds and was off all his medications.*

*Over the next six months, Wayne entered the Second Phase*
*of the program, the health and weight management phase,*
*and continued to use two or three shakes daily, ate six to*
*eight servings of fruits and vegetables, and made sensible*
*low-fat food choices. His weight stabilized at 172.5 pounds,*
*down 147.5 pounds, an excellent body weight for his large*
*frame.*

Following is Wayne's weekly summary chart. Wayne got off to a
fast start with a weight loss of 13 pounds in the first week. Although he consumed less than the dietary minimums for
shakes, entrées, fruits, and vegetables about 25 percent of the
time, he only went off the diet three days during the fourteen
weeks. As a result, Wayne lost 78 pounds in fourteen weeks and
lost 106 pounds after twenty weeks.

**BEGINNING DATE: JUNE 7**
**BEGINNING WEIGHT: 320**

| WEEK | SHAKES | ENTRÉES | FRUITS/ VEGETABLES | BARS | ON THE DIET* | CONSUMED SEFV** | PHYSICAL ACTIVITY | WEIGHT |
|---|---|---|---|---|---|---|---|---|
| 1 | 21 | 14 | 31 | 0 | 7 | 6 | 2585 | 307 |
| 2 | 20 | 14 | 31 | 0 | 4 | 4 | 3580 | 298 |
| 3 | 22 | 14 | 36 | 0 | 7 | 7 | 3180 | 292.5 |
| 4 | 18 | 14 | 41 | 0 | 7 | 5 | 1480 | 288.5 |
| 5 | 23 | 14 | 51 | 0 | 7 | 7 | 3130 | 283.5 |
| 6 | 20 | 14 | 43 | 0 | 7 | 5 | 3130 | 277.5 |
| 7 | 23 | 14 | 29 | 0 | 7 | 7 | 2840 | 274 |
| 8 | 19 | 12 | 43 | 0 | 7 | 3 | 3300 | 269 |
| 9 | 23 | 14 | 49 | 0 | 7 | 7 | 3080 | 264 |
| 10 | 21 | 14 | 41 | 0 | 7 | 5 | 3300 | 258.5 |
| 11 | 19 | 14 | 32 | 0 | 7 | 3 | 3080 | 254 |
| 12 | 19 | 14 | 63 | 0 | 7 | 4 | 3300 | 252.5 |
| 13 | 21 | 14 | 59 | 0 | 7 | 5 | 3580 | 248.5 |
| 14 | 22 | 14 | 45 | 0 | 7 | 4 | 3300 | 242 |

*Consumed only meal replacements, bars, fruits, and vegetables and no other caloric items
**Consumed at least three shakes, two entrées, and five fruits and vegetables

As an engineer, Wayne excelled at Excel spreadsheets (sorry, I couldn't resist the pun), and meticulously filled these out daily. Even though he did not follow the diet perfectly, records helped him keep his feet to the fire and solve problems. On several occasions, especially as he was nearing the end of the First Phase, Wayne increased his intake of fruits and vegetables to help keep him from going off the diet. Even when eating as much as nine servings of fruits and vegetables daily, Wayne still lost weight every week, averaging a 4.3-pound loss weekly after his initial 13-pound loss the first week.

## Is There a Problem?

Recordkeeping helps us identify other types of changes that could aid our weight loss. As I approached my goal weight, I noticed my weight loss was slowing down. When I realized this, I was able to think about what I was doing and realized I was choosing higher-calorie fruits (bananas) and vegetables (beans). To get back into the success cycle, I practiced adding more volume and variety by having more volume in my shakes, using lower-calorie fruits (strawberries) in my shakes, and choosing lower-calorie vegetables (carrots, celery, cherry tomatoes, and red peppers).

Rob was a busy dentist who was eating three bars daily to keep him going. Use of bars is recommended for emergencies, when entrées or shakes are not possible, and for occasional enjoyment. Looking at Rob's records, we decided that the three bars he was having (providing a total of 480 calories) was slowing down his weight loss. We agreed that maybe having an entrée, like Healthy Choice Country Herb Chicken (270 calories) instead of two bars in the afternoon might keep him going just as well. He tried that and was pleased with how he felt. He lost an extra half pound the next week because of this simple change.

Susan had bad knees and was frustrated because she could not do the walking she had always enjoyed. She was only burning 550 calories per week. We recommended that she explore water aerobics at her nearby YMCA. She found that she could do three classes per week without major discomfort from her knees. With our counseling and advice from the trainer at the YMCA, she began doing exercises using dumbbells three days weekly. She could do this while watching the evening news. We calculated that she was burning about 300 calories three times weekly with water aerobics (900 calories) and about 200 calories three times weekly with her weight training (600 calories). She was pleased and excited when she brought in her records showing 2,050 calories of physical activity for the week. Furthermore, she lost an extra pound that week. The physical activities energized her, and she could follow the diet more carefully. We give you more tips about different challenges and how to meet them in chapter 9. Careful recordkeeping helps you plan better and stay in the success cycle.

# A Powerful Tool

As one of the Six Keys of the Simple Diet, recordkeeping is a powerful tool for both successful weight loss and long-term weight management. Tracking your progress as you lose weight will help you stay on the diet. It will keep you motivated and show you how far you've come. It provides information that will allow you to be strategic in overcoming challenges. And it will provide a source of accountability, the last of the Six Keys, which I'll talk about next.

"I can keep accurate records of my intake of shakes, entrées, bars, fruits, and vegetables, as well as my physical activity. I can review my records three times daily and use them to plan for the next part of the day or tomorrow."

# Accountability: Gathering Support and Enlisting Help

8

What is one of *the* most important factors in losing weight? A steady supply of low-calorie foods? Plenty of willpower? Regular exercise? The scientifically proven answer may surprise you: *support*. Being accountable to someone—a supportive or helpful friend or family member—is one of the Six Keys of the Simple Diet.

All of us are more successful in achieving goals if we know we have to report our progress regularly. Although some people prefer to go it alone in their weight-loss journey, most of us do better with a structured system of accountability and personal support.

In group programs, weekly weigh-ins can provide this type of structure and support, but you don't need to enroll in a group to pursue the Simple Diet. Using the information in this chapter, you can create your own system of accountability and support with the help of your doctor and/or others—family, friends, coworkers, or even Internet support groups. And remember, you *have* to enlist the help of your doctor to follow you medically and help you adjust any obesity-related medications you may be taking.

Having at least one support person can help keep you on the right track. If you know your friend is going to ask tomorrow how you did today, you might—even when they are not present—think twice about eating foods that aren't part of your diet plan. In this respect, your support person is like Jiminy Cricket sitting on your shoulder, reminding you of the better course of action. But your support person can also accompany you on your journey literally. For example, many people find that if they have someone to walk with, they are much more likely to get out and walk every day. No one wants to disappoint a friend who's altered his or her schedule to walk with you some early morning. Your support person can also be an ear to listen to your weight-loss successes and failures, help you problem-solve the inevitable challenges of weight loss, and keep you motivated on difficult days.

## Building a Support Network

*Amanda was a twenty-two-year-old graduate student who had completed her BS degree in elementary education and was working on her master's degree and substitute teaching. She had moved home after graduating from college. Her initial weight was 215 pounds, with a height of five feet six inches.*

*Amanda was in good general health, but her primary care physician had expressed concern about her weight and high*

*LDL (bad-guy) cholesterol value of 147 mg/dl. Because of her strong family history of heart disease, this abnormal lab value had triggered her decision to make a serious commitment to weight loss. She was aware that this LDL cholesterol elevation increased her risk for heart attack by 50 percent.*

*Amanda's mother also needed to lose a few pounds and decided to partner with her in this venture. Amanda and her mother arranged to walk together and logged an average of three miles daily throughout the program. Each day they reviewed their successes on the diet from the previous day.*

*Amanda followed the recommendations of using a minimum of three shakes, two entrées, and five fruits and vegetables daily and lost 20 pounds in ten weeks. During spring break, she went on a seven-day cruise with friends and lost (yes, lost) another 5 pounds during her vacation!*

*Amanda lost 49 pounds in 27 weeks. She then entered the Second Phase, the health and weight management phase of the program. Her LDL cholesterol was 97 mg/dl, down fifty points! This drop in weight and cholesterol level greatly lowered her risk for heart attack. She lost another 16 pounds in ten weeks during the Second Phase to reach her goal of 150 pounds.*

Research indicates that the most helpful support partners are those who are on their own weight-loss journeys. Mother and daughter Helen and Pam (chapter 2) as well as Amanda and Cathy (in the following pages) illustrate the synergy of family members working together in their weight-loss efforts. However, you may not have a family member or friend who is poised to enter a weight-loss venture with you at present. It is important for you to try to find a person or group who can support you and help you stay on track as you lose weight. Choose people who will reinforce your positive behaviors and provide encouragement and understanding. An ideal support group might include role models, others who have successfully made the same journey. Find people who encourage self-acceptance and are willing to provide an outlet for you to discuss emotional issues that sometimes surface during weight loss.

Family members can provide a valuable source of support, especially if they also need to lose weight and will go on the Simple Diet with you. Many of my patients have been family members working together on the diet, but even if family members aren't using the Simple Diet, they can still help by exercising with you and not bringing tempting, high-fat foods like chips or ice cream that trigger overeating into the house.

Your spouse can also be a valuable source of support. Sometimes both spouses will tackle weight loss together, while other times one spouse works on weight loss while the other provides encouragement and support. Often when one spouse loses weight, the other will be inspired to lose, too.

*Cathy, a fifty-four-year-old homemaker, and her husband both wanted to lose more than 100 pounds. Her husband enrolled in the program and lost 105 pounds in seven months. Cathy decided to follow the Simple Diet at home without coming to the clinic. She and her husband consumed meal replacements, fruits, and vegetables and walked together. As her husband learned that using more than five meal replacements per day helped him avoid hunger, she also started using more than five meal replacements daily. We do*

> *not have detailed records of Cathy's physical activity, but she*
> *did share that she has stopped all blood pressure and arthritis*
> *medicine and feels wonderful. Over twenty-six weeks, she lost*
> *111 pounds and continues to lose weight with her husband,*
> *who is in the Second Phase of the program.*

A family member or spouse is not always the best choice for support. Some people find that partnering with their spouse for weight loss just doesn't work, particularly if emotional issues are involved. Spouses or family members can also wind up interfering with your weight loss, sometimes without even realizing it. They might suggest going out to eat at a restaurant where many tempting desserts are available, or bring home the leftover coffee cake from work. Sometimes family members feel threatened by or jealous of your weight loss and intentionally try to sabotage your efforts.

In lieu of a family member, a friend, a coworker, or an Internet support group may be viable options for support and accountability. The many weight-loss forums on the Internet give users the opportunity to trade ideas, discuss successes and setbacks, and connect with others who face similar challenges. Below are just a few of the many helpful Internet weight-loss forums and sites. Appendix 8.1, Features of Some Weight-Loss Websites, gives more detailed information on these sites and what features each site offers.

- sparkpeople.com
- startyourdiet.com
- livestrong.com
- fatsecret.com

- everydayhealth.com
- caloriecount.about.com
- eatthis.com

Many of my family members are on Facebook. If you are engaged in some form of social media, ask your online friends about whether they might be interested in working with you. You might find a number of people who would be eager to do this. It's easy to use e-mail or one of the social networking options to send out regular reports and get their encouraging comments as you make progress. At our website, www.andersonsimplediet .com, we also maintain an interactive blog to help answer your questions.

Try to check in with a support person at least weekly. Tell him or her how you are doing with all aspects of the program, including whether or not you are staying on the Simple Diet, how much physical activity you are doing, and whether you are getting at least the minimum recommended servings of shakes, entrées, fruits, and vegetables. Share with them any challenges you are confronting, or if you had a particularly rough day. Ask them to help you problem-solve anything that is not working well for you. Finally, suggest specific ways that they can help you, such as going to the gym with you or rearranging the refrigerator so fruits and vegetables are front and center.

## Enlisting Your Doctor's Help

You will also need the help of your own doctor before you even start this program. Acting as coaches, encouraging you as you make positive changes in your weight and health, and helping you meet challenges, your doctor and his or her health care team can be a valuable source of ongoing accountability and support.

However, you must talk to your doctor *before* you start the Simple Diet, and you may need to return for medical monitoring and follow-up for your own safety and health. My research shows that 97 percent of people with severe obesity have at least one obesity-related condition (and usually more), like high blood pressure, diabetes, or high cholesterol, and 74 percent take medications for those conditions.[37] Many individuals with even mild or moderate obesity are taking medications for obesity-related problems. As people lose excess weight under this program, two out of three are able to discontinue their medications—a gradual process that requires medical monitoring and physician guidance.

It's important to choose a doctor who has experience in helping people lose weight, who is supportive, and who is truly interested in partnering with you to help you in this process. Establish a regular check-in schedule with your doctor or one of his staff members, and return for regular check-ins as recommended by your doctor or if problems arise. Your doctor can:

- tell you if it's safe for you to undertake the Simple Diet;
- tell you how to adjust your medications as you lose weight;
- identify medical risks;
- provide ongoing medical monitoring and follow-up; and
- serve as a source of support and accountability.

# Talking with Your Doctor

Your doctor will probably appreciate if you bring a list of important information to your appointment so he or she can more quickly assess your situation and suitability for starting the Simple Diet.

**Family health history (mother, father, siblings, aunts, uncles, grandparents) of any of the following problems:**

- Diabetes
- Heart disease
- Strokes
- High blood pressure
- Any other important problems

**Personal health history:**

- Diabetes, gestational diabetes, or borderline blood glucose results in the past
- Heart attack, chest pain, recent stress test
- Prior stroke or transient ischemic attack (TIA)
- High blood pressure (bring in recent blood pressure results if you measure your own blood pressure)
- Snoring, daytime sleeping, or other symptoms of sleep apnea
- Any other important problems

**Medications:**

- List all prescription and nonprescription medications, such as aspirin

**Past weight-loss attempts:**

- List year, program or diet, pounds lost

**Current level of physical activity:**

- Regular walking
- Jogging, exercise bike, other cardio and aerobic activities
- Visits to the gym
- Weight lifting
- Other activities

**Barriers to weight loss:**

- Home environment where another person will not be agreeable to limiting visibility and availability of tempting high-fat foods
- Work or travel schedule that will present challenges in doing physical activity and obtaining meal replacements, fruits, and vegetables
- Work environment that is loaded with problem foods
- Social schedule that includes many meals away from home
- Other barriers

**Barriers to physical activity:**

- Arthritis or other challenges that limit walking and other physical activities
- Time availability
- Other barriers

If your doctor is not familiar with the Simple Diet, you may want to bring a copy of this book with you at your first visit so he or she can understand the Six Keys of the program and what you will be trying to accomplish. Appendix 8.2, Summary of the Simple Diet for Your Doctor, gives a brief summary of the Simple Diet to share with your doctor, as well as some notes about medical supervision needed on this diet.

# Special Medical Considerations

The Simple Diet is not for women who are pregnant or breast-feeding. Discontinue the diet immediately and tell your doctor if you become pregnant. The Simple Diet is intended for adults only. Although I have treated several hundred adolescents with the Simple Diet and done research in this area, this diet should only be used by teenagers under strict medical supervision.

Certain medical conditions require special consideration when undergoing any weight-loss program.

**If you have high blood pressure, you should discuss these things with your doctor:**

- How often you should monitor your blood pressure yourself
- What changes you should make in your blood pressure medications
- How often you will need to go into the office for monitoring
- Symptoms and signs of low blood pressure and when you should contact the office

If you have cerebrovascular disease—such as a recent stroke or transient ischemic attack (TIA)—you need to avoid low blood pressure. We do not recommend that you start on the diet until you have been stable for at least one month after this event. You should discuss the diet with your doctor and be alert to dizziness when you stand up suddenly or when you get out of bed. Talk to your doctor about any blood pressure medicines you are taking and plan to monitor your own blood pressure.

**If you have diabetes, you should discuss these things with your doctor:**

- How often you need to measure your blood glucose values while on the Simple Diet
- How much you should reduce your insulin dose when you start the diet
- How you should alter your doses of other diabetes medications when starting the diet
- How often you need to be seen by your doctor
- Blood glucose values or symptoms that should prompt you to contact your doctor

If you have diabetes, you should be aware that decreasing your calorie intake will have a dramatic effect on your blood glucose values. It is imperative for you to consult your doctor before starting the diet. I have treated over a thousand diabetic patients with the Simple Diet and other intensive weight-loss programs, but of course, this is my area of medical specialization and research interest. In type 2 diabetes, we usually reduce insulin doses and oral medication doses by about 80 percent during the diet and discontinue most diabetes medications in more than 70 percent of our patients. Of course, our endocrinology team has to monitor these changes closely and be available to coach the patient so they avoid hypoglycemic reactions.

**You should also talk to your doctor if you have any of the following conditions:**

- Recent thrombophlebitis; dehydration from insufficient fluid intake can aggravate this problem
- Severe kidney disease; I have treated many people with severe kidney disease safely, but they require careful medical monitoring
- Severe liver disease; I have treated many patients with severe liver disease (including those who were on the waiting list for liver transplants), but again, they required careful medical monitoring

## Medication Considerations

If you are on certain medicines, your doctor may need to monitor you and adjust doses as needed.

- **Diuretics:** If you are taking a diuretic such as hydrochlorothiazide, you should see your doctor for recommendations. Because your meal replacements are low in sodium, people usually get rid of some extra body water when they go on the diet. For this reason, we usually discontinue diuretics when people start the diet. If you have a lot of edema—especially swelling of your ankles—or have a history of congestive heart failure, you should discuss this with your primary care provider.
- **Coumadin:** If you are taking this blood thinner, your primary care provider will want to monitor your prothrombin to see if changes in doses are required.

- **Lithium:** If you are taking lithium, you should discuss the diet with your psychiatrist managing this drug. Weekly blood levels for lithium, sodium, and potassium may be required. Also, you should drink at least three quarts of water daily.
- **Trileptal:** This drug can cause dangerously low levels of serum sodium. We do not recommend that you start on the diet without weekly monitoring by your treating physician.

# Possible Side Effects

Most people feel great and have more energy on the Simple Diet than before they started the plan. The need for medication drops, and many medical issues—such as diabetes, high blood pressure, or high blood cholesterol levels—are reversed.

The most common side effects we have seen in our medically supervised patients using meal replacements only, with no fruits or vegetables, include constipation, dizziness, headaches, diarrhea, fatigue, flatulence, abdominal pain, and nausea. Side effects are much less common when you add fruits and vegetables.

However, when you lose weight rapidly, you may experience a short bout of some of these symptoms:

**Gastrointestinal symptoms:** Any big change in dietary practices can result in gastrointestinal complaints, such as abdominal discomfort, nausea, flatulence, diarrhea, or constipation.

Most adults in the United States do not consume five servings of fruits and vegetables daily, and the increased fiber and bulk in these, called for in the Simple Diet, can cause transient abdominal discomfort and more frequent bowel movements. Abdominal discomfort and diarrhea usually clear up in a few days to a few weeks. Nausea can be related to lactose intolerance (see below) or timing and volume of the shakes. If you develop constipation, you should begin using one dose of psyllium (Metamucil) once or twice daily.

**Lactose intolerance:** If you have documented lactose intolerance—nausea, abdominal discomfort, diarrhea—after using dairy products, you should select a milk-free shake (such as Revival Soy shakes). You may be able to use other shakes containing lactose if you use Lactaid before consuming them.

**Light-headedness and dizziness:** Light-headedness and dizziness can be due to inadequate fluid intake or low blood pressure. If you get dizzy when you stand up suddenly or when you get out of bed, this may be related to low blood pressure, especially if you are taking blood pressure medicine. Check your blood pressure at a local pharmacy, and schedule an appointment with your primary care physician if your blood pressure is below 110 systolic over 70 diastolic.

If you are not on blood pressure medicine, dizziness is likely related to not drinking enough fluids. Remember, the goal is to drink a minimum of eight glasses (64 oz.) of noncaloric fluid per day. If you are not on blood pressure medicine, increase your fluid intake to at least twelve glasses of noncaloric fluid daily and add one cup of half-strength, low-fat bouillon twice daily. Some antianxiety and antidepressant medications could also contribute to dizziness. Check with your doctor if dizziness persists.

**Headaches:** The Simple Diet may initially be accompanied by mild headaches just because of reduced calorie intake. Eating more frequently usually alleviates headaches. When I seriously restrict my calories, I get mild headaches and slight fatigue that decrease as I adjust to the diet. The stress of the diet may precipitate more frequent migraine headaches for migraine sufferers, but after a few weeks on the diet, the migraine attacks are usually less frequent than before starting the diet.

**Fatigue:** Some individuals experience slight fatigue or decreased energy after starting the diet. This usually abates after two to three weeks. Having meals or snacks every three hours during the day diminishes these symptoms. The good news is that most people have more energy with the Simple Diet.

**Hair loss:** Loss of hair occurs occasionally after weight losses of 30 to 50 pounds. This is not due to nutritional deficiencies, but simply to the stress that weight loss puts on your body. Other types of stress can also cause hair loss. Over my many years of helping patients lose weight, I have never seen an individual who had substantial hair loss, and in all people with mild hair loss, losses reversed and hair patterns returned to baseline after the person entered the Second Phase of the plan and started eating a weight-maintaining diet.

**Gallbladder disease:** Gallstones and gallbladder disease are severalfold higher in overweight individuals than in slender individuals. About one-third of severely obese individuals develop gallstones.

The changes in diet associated with weight loss may cause development of symptomatic gallstones in persons who already have a tendency to develop gallbladder disease. About 1 percent of the patients I have treated developed symptomatic gallbladder disease while on the diet or within six months after completing the weight-loss phase.

If you have a history of gallbladder disease, discuss the diet with your primary care provider. Actigall, 300 mg twice daily, greatly decreases the risk of developing gallstones; we do not use it routinely, but do prescribe it when people have a prior history of gallbladder disease or develop symptoms while on the diet. Discuss this issue with your primary care provider if you have concerns.

# Going It Alone

As previously discussed, anyone embarking on the Simple Diet will need the help of his or her doctor to monitor any medications or medical conditions. Other than that, you may be one of those people who prefer to work on losing weight by yourself. Not everyone wants or needs support. Some people like to exercise with a partner to keep them going and motivated to keep showing up. Others prefer to walk alone. Personally, I like to use my time walking for reflection and meditation.

If you do choose to go it alone, you'll need to provide your own system of accountability and check in with your doctor regularly. Your recordkeeping takes on even greater importance. Keep your daily progress and weekly summary charts as reviewed in chapter 7. Weigh yourself at least weekly and write down your weights on your weekly summary chart. Bring your charts with you when it's time to check in with your doctor.

*Aaron, a twenty-six-year-old graduate student, was five feet eleven inches tall and weighed 290 pounds. He was a self-assured young man and very personable. Aaron decided he could follow the Simple Diet on his own. He started using three shakes and two entrées along with at least five servings of fruits and vegetables daily. After about six months on the plan, our receptionist asked him how he was doing. He told her he'd lost over 100 pounds using the general guidelines of the Simple Diet.*

# A Final Checklist

Now that we've talked about accountability and support, we've finished explaining the Six Keys of the Simple Diet. You are ready to start on the First Phase, the intensive weight-loss phase. Use the checklist below to be sure you have everything ready.

### Checklist for Starting the Simple Diet
❏ Obtained your doctor's permission to start the diet.
❏ Talked with your doctor about any medications you are on.
❏ Purchased at least a week's worth of shakes, entrées, fruits, and vegetables.
❏ Made your kitchen user-friendly by having meal replacements, fruits, and vegetables readily accessible.
❏ Precut fruits and vegetables so they are quick and easy to eat or prepare.
❏ Own a good quality blender for making a variety of delicious shakes and variations.

- ❑ Have the needed containers and supplies to take meal replacements with you or make them at work.
- ❑ Printed out daily progress and weekly summary charts to keep a written record of your success.
- ❑ Enlisted the help of your doctor and, if desired, family members, friends, and coworkers.
- ❑ Thought about your weight-loss goals and motivators for losing weight.
- ❑ Thought about potential obstacles to staying on the diet or increasing physical activity and developed a plan to overcome them.
- ❑ Own a good pair of walking shoes or other appropriate exercise clothes and equipment.
- ❑ Planned how you will increase your physical activity to at least 2,000 calories weekly.

In the remaining chapters, we'll talk about how to deal with challenges in the First Phase, how to transition into the Second Phase, and how to take charge of your health for life.

"I can review my Simple Diet

plans with my doctor and share

my progress toward

my goals with an affirming

support person."

# If Your Weight Loss Slows: Boosting Weight Loss and Meeting Challenges

Keith, a forty-four-year-old health insurance executive, recently learned that his blood cholesterol level was high (his LDL cholesterol, the bad kind of cholesterol, was 133 mg/dl). Working in the health care business and with a father who died at age fifty-six from a heart attack, Keith knew the consequences of high blood cholesterol. At six feet tall, he weighed in at 227 pounds. With his busy travel schedule, he did not always plan carefully and sometimes found himself without the shakes or entrées he needed. Also, while he could walk thirty miles some weeks, other weeks he only managed to walk four to six miles per week, averaging about ten miles walking per week. Keith was struggling, but with coaching and encouragement, he lost 34 pounds in fifteen weeks. His cholesterol level dropped into the desirable range (LDL cholesterol of 90 mg/dl), and he avoided having to take a statin drug to lower his cholesterol.

Going on a diet is easy, and losing a little weight is easy. Most of us have done it dozens of times. Losing to our goal weight or an ideal weight for health protection is not as easy.

In August 2008, when I decided to get into shape and lose 25 pounds to get back to my high school weight, I thought, "This will not be too difficult; it's only twenty-five pounds." After all, for twenty-five years I had directed what many believe to be one of the best weight-management programs in the world. I just needed to get the meal replacements, stock up on fruits and vegetables, join the YMCA, and start recording my progress. Because I was overweight and not obese, I did not expect to lose four to eight pounds per week, but would have been happy with two or three pounds per week.

Well, I lost three pounds the first week and then two pounds the next—and then one pound the next week! During the next six months of achieving my health-promoting weight, I learned many lessons about being successful, and also about not being successful. My experience is similar to that of many of my patients.

In this chapter, I want to help readers who are struggling. What do you do when your weight loss slows or goes the wrong way? What happens if you find yourself off the plan? What if you feel burned out, or feel like you're hitting the wall? This chapter will give you ideas to help you sustain weight loss and meet challenges.

## Some of Us Have to Work Harder at Weight Loss Than Others

My own physician lost more than 30 pounds about ten years ago. When I complimented him on maintaining a slender build, he confided, "But it's hard, Jim; I have to work at it every day."

Research shows that overweight or obese individuals have more trouble maintaining their weight at a health-promoting level than do people who were never overweight. Like my own doctor and me, these individuals will need to work harder at weight loss.

Genetic factors, some lifelong ingrained lifestyle habits, decreased metabolism rates, changes in appetite or satiety hormones, and other factors all play a role in this inequity. Some of us are hyperkinetic, even without caffeine or nicotine, while others are more placid. Some, like me, are volume eaters, while others, like my slender wife, are nibblers. Like Kenny Rogers suggests in his song "The Gambler," we all need to play the hand we're dealt, and every hand can be a winner.

To win by losing, we need to monitor our weights and exercise habits, commit nearly three hundred minutes weekly to physical activity and fitness, eat more fruits and vegetables, become fat detectives and minimize all types of fat intake, limit the intake of foods with added caloric sweeteners, decrease exposure to fast foods, and eat a smaller variety of foods than many slender individuals.

## We Don't All Lose at the Same Rate

Rates of weight loss vary greatly from person to person. Your ability to lose weight depends largely on your starting body weight, metabolic rate, level of physical activity, and the total number of calories you consume.

If you weigh 150 pounds, you will lose weight more slowly than a person who weighs 250 pounds. If you are close to your health-promoting weight, you will lose weight more slowly than people who are 50 pounds or more overweight. If you are an older individual, your metabolic rate may be slower than that of a younger individual, slowing your weight loss.

For reasons not fully understood, the rate at which people lose weight with diets slows down over time. The Simple Diet is no exception. The figure below tracks the weight of twenty-two individuals on the Simple Diet. They had an average starting weight of 220 pounds and lost an average of 12 pounds at four weeks, 20 pounds at eight weeks, 26 pounds at twelve weeks, and 30 pounds at sixteen weeks. Thus, for each successive four-week period, these individuals lost an average of 12, 8, 6, and 4 pounds.[38]

**Average Weight Losses**

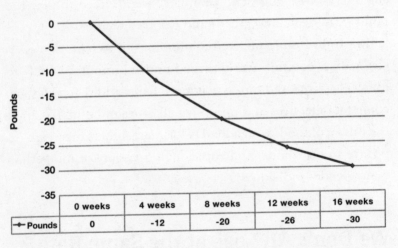

| | 0 weeks | 4 weeks | 8 weeks | 12 weeks | 16 weeks |
|---|---|---|---|---|---|
| Pounds | 0 | -12 | -20 | -26 | -30 |

Most individuals on the Simple Diet lose a little more water weight in the first one to three weeks after starting the plan than in the following weeks. Changes in water weight at different points in the weight-loss journey can also mask changes in actual body fat lost. If your weight loss slows down too much, however, it's easy to become discouraged.

Some people, like Keith, may struggle to stick with certain elements of the Simple Diet, slowing their rate of weight loss. Other people think they are carefully following the plan but, on close scrutiny, are consuming hidden calories from sources they were not aware of. Still other people struggle with painstakingly slow weight loss despite complete compliance with the plan and may need to boost their weight loss by emphasizing the lowest-calorie choices of meal replacements, fruits, and vegetables, and by adding volume to their diet.

The table below lists the absolute *minimum* four-week weight losses individuals at different weights should expect to continue to achieve after starting the Simple Diet. If your weight is not dropping at this minimum rate, we want to help you look carefully at how you can boost your weight loss and meet any challenges you may have to sticking with the plan.

| WEIGHT RANGE | FOUR-WEEK WEIGHT LOSS |
| --- | --- |
| <150 pounds | 2 pounds |
| 150–174 pounds | 3 pounds |
| 175–199 pounds | 4 pounds |
| 200–249 pounds | 6 pounds |
| 250–299 pounds | 8 pounds |
| 300–399 pounds | 12 pounds |
| 400 pounds or more | 16 pounds |

# Give Yourself Some Credit

Although I know it's disappointing and discouraging when you are not losing weight as fast as you would like, try to first focus on all the things you are doing right. You are reading this book, are using meal replacements, fruits, and vegetables, and have increased your physical activity level. Give yourself credit for all these positive changes you have made.

Some parts of the Simple Diet may not have fallen into place for you. Are you having trouble keeping good records of your food intake and physical activity? Maybe you are having trouble sticking with the plan. Are you having a problem getting in the minimum number of meal replacements or fruits and vegetables? Or maybe you are having hunger pangs, slight headaches, or less energy. Let's talk about these.

## Take a Close Look at Your Records

The first step in meeting weight-loss challenges is to diligently keep your records and use them to help you problem-solve. You may believe you're following the Simple Diet, but in reality, you could be missing something important.

I have walked through this with many people. I often start the conversation something like this: "You're doing a good job. Your physical activity is higher and you're eating fruits and vegetables. We may be having a numbers problem. Let's see if your records can help us understand why you're not losing weight as fast as we would expect." Often when we walk through the day together, we discover that calories are creeping in that the individual was not really conscious of.

For example, one of my patients ordered a large regular coffee from the coffee shop each day, but he didn't account for the fact that the "regular coffee" in this shop had cream and sugar already added. Another very bright attorney drank ten cups of coffee daily and always added two creamers to each cup. This was such a habit for her that it somehow never registered that it was adding 1,420 calories per day to her diet (71 calories per creamer packet times twenty packets per day). When we reviewed her daily activities and I asked if she added cream or sugar to her coffee, she hit her forehead with her palm and exclaimed, "Duh! How many calories are in a coffee creamer?"

A chef patient indicated that he did not taste while cooking, so we asked him to wear a surgical mask the next day at work. Within a few minutes, the mask was so covered in small unconscious "tastes" that he had to take it off.

Sometimes people compartmentalize things and really do not remember them. Just as sleepwalkers don't remember sleepwalking, some people eat during the day or at night and are not fully aware of it. Patients tell me that they find Snickers bar wrappers under the seat of the car and they don't remember buying them or eating them. I believe that eating surreptitiously is so painful for some individuals that they suppress or compartmentalize the episodes.

So if you are not losing weight like you expect to, it is possible that you may be going off the plan without realizing it. The best way to avoid this is to revisit the Six Keys to Intensive Weight Loss (chapter 3). Using three shakes and two entrées, eating five or more servings of fruits and vegetables, drinking at least eight glasses of water, and adding volume will all fill you up and reduce hunger, lessening your inclination to go off the diet. When you exercise, you'll feel better and will be more likely to sustain that feeling by staying on the diet. Keeping records will help you be more aware of your choices and help you stay on the diet. Finally, being accountable to someone will give you support and encouragement to keep on the diet and keep going.

# Four Strategies to Boost Your Weight Loss

Even the most diligent dieters will see their weight loss slow down, but here are some strategies for keeping weight loss steady. These four strategies will help you sustain your weight loss and overcome challenges.

- Consume at least three shakes, two entrées, and five servings of fruits and vegetables (SEFV).
- Stay on the diet—consume SEFV, meet your physical activity goals, keep records, and check in with someone to establish accountability.
- Eat more—yes, that's right, more! More shakes, entrées, fruits, and vegetables.
- Add more variety and more volume.

## Consuming the Recommended Servings of Shakes, Entrées, Fruits, and Vegetables

Meeting the recommended three shakes, two entrées, and five servings of fruits and vegetables is the foundation of the Simple Diet. Consuming *at least* the recommended servings meets your daily minimum for protein, provides you with a lot of food to eat, and helps you avoid other higher-calorie off-diet foods.

Protein is the most satiating nutrient in the diet. Eating more protein gives you a sense of satisfaction and diminishes hunger. Further, adding at least five servings of fruits and vegetables to the diet gives you more to chew on, curbs hunger, and adds nutrition. My experience indicates that when people do not consume the minimum required number of shakes and entrées, they experience side effects and fall off the wagon much sooner that those who consume the recommended servings.

Our research documents that consuming *at least* the recommended servings of meal replacements and fruits and vegetables is essential for safety and success with weight loss.[39] Some people have tried to take four meal replacements instead of five to shave off calories, but, almost always, they wind up finding more calories by eating other higher-calorie foods that are not on the plan. So our number-one recommendation for successful weight loss: Consume the recommended servings of shakes, entrées, fruits, and vegetables!

# Staying On the Diet

The greatest challenge for most people on the Simple Diet is to avoid food that is not on the diet plan. During the weight-loss phase, this is extremely important. This is the biggest problem I had while in the First Phase. Since I am such an "expert," I try to redefine what is on the plan! When I go to Starbucks with my children and grandchildren, I decide the soy latte is on the diet—NOT! When we stop at a nice ice-cream shop, I decide that fruit sorbet is a serving of fruit—NOT! When we go to a restaurant, while a baked potato with salt and pepper is on the plan, garlic mashed potatoes with plenty of butter are NOT!

The guidelines we provide for staying on the diet are not draconian, but they do not give you carte blanche to make choices of items that obviously are much higher in fat and calories than this carefully crafted program recommends. So if you want to lose weight, stick with the plan: shakes, entrées, fruits, and vegetables.

However, it is nearly impossible for many people to never go off the plan. The big problem is not having the first few chips; it's realizing, once you've had those first few chips, that you have gone off the plan and therefore thinking that you might as well enjoy yourself, rationalizing that you have already blown the diet for the day.

When you accidentally fall off the wagon, get back on immediately. The indiscretion probably represents fewer than 50 calories, but when you give yourself permission to "enjoy yourself," you may accumulate ten, twenty, even thirty times that amount. And while you're "enjoying yourself," you may decide that you can skip your physical activity for the day and add insult to injury.

In my personal experience with hundreds of patients I have helped to lose weight, when people feel they have more flexibility and go off the plan because they don't have so much weight to lose, they can quickly derail their progress. Stay on the diet. Consume the recommended minimum servings of shakes, entrées, fruits, and vegetables; get in your 2,000 calories of physical activity; keep records; and be accountable to someone. Sticking with the plan is indispensable for your long-term weight-loss success.

# Eating More—More Meal Replacements, Fruits, and Vegetables

*Gloria was a thirty-eight-year-old MRI technician who, at five feet three inches tall, weighed in at 170 pounds. While she was barely in the obese category, she was concerned about her overweight state and her slightly high LDL cholesterol. She wanted to be able to keep up with her soccer-playing eleven-year-old daughter. As a working mother who did some overtime, she was attracted to the "no decision" aspects of the diet and its convenience. Using at least three shakes and two entrées as well as five to six fruit and vegetable servings per day, she lost weight slowly but steadily. She was careful to stick with the plan, but often found herself hungry or craving something more. To combat this, she consumed more shakes, entrées, fruits, and vegetables than the recommended minimum. Over twenty-four weeks, she lost 35 pounds and her LDL cholesterol dropped 30 points. Her daughter, who was becoming weight-conscious herself, complimented her mother on her new figure.*

Many of our most successful patients practice the eating-more strategy to sustain their weight loss. A recent comparison of 534 patients in Health Management Resources clinic programs showed that those patients using seven to eight shakes and entrées daily were losing three times more weight than those using only five to six shakes and entrées per day.[40]

Most individuals benefit from increasing their intake of shakes and entrées if their weight loss is less than expected. Using more shakes and entrées than the minimum and consuming more than five servings of fruits and vegetables will help you stay on the plan and curb hunger that could set you up to go off the plan with higher-calorie foods such as chips or sweets.

Most people develop a "less is better" mentality while dieting. They try to eat *less* often, put *less* food on their plates, and eat *fewer* calories. Unfortunately, it's a near certainty that if you've tried this for even a few days or a week, you've begun to run out of gas. But at this point, because you've deprived yourself you may tell yourself that you have a big negative calorie deposit "in the bank" and can have anything you want. In short order, you've eaten back all you sacrificed for and then some.

Let's say you are a 200-pound woman. You need about 2,200 calories to sustain this weight if you are a couch potato. Let's say you do fine on three shakes, two entrées, and five servings of fruits and vegetables; you should lose about 2.5 pounds per week.

But, if you are struggling with hunger, you could go up to eight shakes or entrées and ten servings of fruits and vegetables and *still* lose one pound per week! So if you are having trouble with gnawing hunger or having a slight headache from the lack of calories, eat more Simple Diet–approved foods to relieve these problems and allow you to continue your successful weight loss.

## Pump Up the Volume!

*Barbara was a fifty-one-year-old CPA with a height of five feet three inches and a weight of 200 pounds. She had a litany of medical problems, including diabetes, high blood cholesterol, arthritis, swelling of the ankles, and indigestion. She was taking ten prescription medications and six over-the-counter medications daily. She entered the program enthusiastically and, like most accountants, was a methodical record keeper.*

*With encouragement and coaching, Barbara lost 32 pounds in twenty-four weeks and continued to lose weight for another eight weeks. Her blood glucose and cholesterol values improved dramatically, and she was able to discontinue her diabetes drug and the statin drug for cholesterol. When her weight reached 170 and below, Barbara found she needed to choose lower-calorie entrées and lower-calorie fruits and vegetables to help sustain her weight loss, but she also still wanted to be satisfied and not experience hunger. She found that she could trade in a serving of corn for a large green salad, cut calories, and feel fuller. She also started adding extra liquid to her shakes for extra volume. After thirty-two weeks on the program, she entered the health and weight management phase and achieved her weight goal of getting under 155 pounds.*

Persons who weigh less than 180 pounds or are getting close to their goal weight may need to focus on more volume in their shakes and fewer calories in their entrées, fruits, and vegetables. Choosing carrots, celery, cherry tomatoes, green beans, red pepper strips, or spinach instead of garbanzo beans, corn, peas, and potatoes will help you lose an extra half a pound in a week. For fruits, choose melon, peaches, strawberries, and tangerines, with fewer servings of bananas and cherries.

Extensive research indicates that high-volume, low-calorie foods have major advantages for weight loss and long-term weight management. Drinking a glass of water before each meal will give you a sense of fullness and decrease food intake at that meal.

As I worked to get my weight below 160 pounds, I used some of the strategies that we had worked out for Barbara. One of my favorites was using high-volume shakes. While writing this, I am sipping on a root beer–strawberry shake that has 160 calories in 22-ounce volume (7.3 calories per ounce).

## Root Beer–Strawberry Shake

8 oz. cold diet root beer

8 oz. chilled water

1 scoop French Vanilla shake mix (Slim-Fast)

2 packets sweetener

½ packet sugar-free gelatin

4 large frozen strawberries

4 ice cubes

Add the root beer and water to the blender and blend briefly on low. Add the shake mix, sweetener, and gelatin and blend again.

Add the strawberries while blending on low. When blended, add the ice cubes one at a time. Blend well on high. Enjoy.

The table below illustrates how you can get your daily shakes and entrées (breakfast, lunch, dinner, and two snacks) in either a low-volume or a high-volume way. The high-volume plan is much more filling than the low-volume one.

| LOW-VOLUME | HIGH-VOLUME |
|---|---|
| 10 oz. Milk Chocolate shake (Special K) and 1 banana | Vanilla Pleasure shake mix (Revival) blended with 16 oz. water and 1 cup strawberries |
| Vanilla shake (Slim-Rite) | 12 oz. Cappuccino Delight shake (Slim-Fast) and 1 peach |
| Pumpkin Squash Ravioli (Healthy Choice) and ½ cup black beans | Creamy Rigatoni with Broccoli & Chicken (Smart Ones), 1 cup red beets, and 1 tangelo |
| 10 oz. Strawberry shake (Special K) | Vanilla shake mix (GNC) blended with 16 oz. water and 1 tsp. dark cocoa |
| Chicken Margherita (Lean Cuisine), 1 cup mashed winter squash, and 10 sweet cherries | Grilled Shrimp Scampi (Gorton's), 2 cups broccoli medley, and 1 orange |
| Total: 3 shakes, 2 entrées, 5 fruits/vegetables 1,501 calories Volume: 23 calories/ounce | Total: 3 shakes, 2 entrées, 6 fruits/vegetables 1,115 calories Volume: 13 calories/ounce |

The low-volume menu provides 1,501 calories in 65 ounces of food (23 calories/oz.) while the high-volume menu provides 1,115 calories in 86 ounces of food (13 calories/oz.). Saving about 400 calories per day allows you to lose almost one more pound per week! And which diet do you think would be more filling for you?

The entrées, fruits, and vegetables used in both menus are

on the diet. But here is another area where you have the power to influence your success level by the choices you make. You can potentially make selections that deliver a total of 400 to 700 fewer calories in these areas. If you weigh less than 180 pounds or are approaching your goal weight, these selections may make a big difference in your weight loss. Note several differences between the menus in the low- and high-volume columns. First, the selection of entrées affects your calorie intake. Acceptable entrées range from 140 to 300 calories. If you select two entrées at 140 to 200 calories, you save about 90 calories, compared with selecting two entrées between 220 to 300 calories.

Second, you can select low-calorie or high-calorie fruits and vegetables. You can select fruits with 33 to 98 calories per serving; potentially you can save 100 calories per day by selecting two low-calorie fruits. You can select vegetables with 17 to 130 calories per serving! Selecting three low-calorie vegetables can save you at least 40 calories per serving or 120 calories for the day. As I approached my goal weight, I was eating eight to ten servings of fruits and vegetables per day; I had the potential of choosing bananas and beans (high-calorie choices) or strawberries and spinach (low-calorie choices). This could amount to a 500-calorie difference in a day. With my weight loss slowing, I chose the lower-calorie fruits and vegetables, because 500 calories a day represents a pound a week!

Again, in general, persons who weigh less than 180 pounds need to focus on more volume in their shakes and fewer calories from their fruits (strawberries instead of bananas) and vegetables (green beans instead of black beans).

The eating-more strategy also includes eating a greater variety of fruits and vegetables. My good friend David Heber, MD, at UCLA wrote the popular book *What Color Is Your Diet?* In it, he summarizes the benefits of getting a wide variety of colors from your fruits and vegetables. In adding this variety, you are bringing an array of potent antioxidants and other health-promoting phytochemicals to the table.

But adding variety also keeps you from getting bored. An apple a day may keep the doctor away, but mixing things up with fresh peaches, plums, berries, melons, whatever is in season, keeps things interesting and your palate entertained. Visit local farmers' markets or produce stores and try different varieties of fruits and vegetables. Don't let yourself get into a rut.

# Identifying Barriers to Weight Loss

Many overweight adults were raised by parents who equated heavy with healthy. Children were encouraged to clean their plates to grow healthy and strong. A skinny child might reflect negatively on parents—"Why don't they feed that child?" So you may have grown up in an environment where hearty eating was encouraged.

Perhaps you have a spouse who is overweight or obese, and the two of you enjoy all-American foods like bacon, sausage, gravy, well-marbled beef, pork chops, ice cream, and apple pie. You might have friends who are also overweight who enjoy having muffins in the mornings and cookies in the afternoons. Like most of society, many of your social events may revolve around food. So since childhood, your environment encouraged you to eat frequently and gave you a taste for high-fat, high-sugar foods. Even if you lose weight, you will still be in this environment.

Many of us learn to link a certain activity with eating and automatically eat whenever we do that activity. Many people eat without thinking while watching television. The myriad food commercials airing between shows do not help matters. Some people develop a habit of eating while reading, not really realizing what they are eating. For others, overeating is a regular part of bridge, bowling, or Bunco night.

Some people are emotional eaters. You may have developed the habit of using food in response to stress (I am guilty as charged!). If you need to unwind after a hard day, food becomes your de-stressor. If you are worried about the budget or a big event coming up, you may overeat to mask your worry.

Many people overeat out of boredom. Food is interesting and gives them something to do and look forward to. Many of us also eat when we are happy, have good news, or have accomplished a goal. Food, then, becomes a reward for us. Identifying elements of your background or environment associated with overeating can help you overcome your own personal barriers to weight loss.

Some individuals were traumatized as children and developed the habit of overeating in response to the trauma. Individuals who were abused, especially girls, may have gained weight to appear less attractive and draw less attention from boys and men. These are serious issues, and I encourage you to get counseling to help you heal from these wounds.

# Confronting Your Challenges

When you anticipate the challenges to staying on the Simple Diet and plan in advance how you will handle these challenges, you set yourself up for success. Here are some of the challenges we've seen in our patients.

## Challenge #1: Keeping records

Keeping written track of your food intake and physical activity is *vital* to successful weight loss. If you are using meal replacements and fruits and vegetables but not always writing them down in a systematic fashion, carry your daily progress chart with you so it is always handy and you can record food and exercise immediately. Take time to tally things up at the end of each day and each week, and these records will become very useful tools for you to chart your progress and spot weak points, along with celebrating milestones.

In treating thousands of patients, I do not recall anyone who has lost substantial weight without keeping written records of food intake and physical activity. When we were in school, our graded papers and report cards kept us motivated and helped us identify areas where we needed more work. Also, our parents and teachers used this information to help and encourage us. Likewise, keeping daily and weekly progress charts while on the Simple Diet makes you feel good about your progress and helps you identify plans to continue your weight management success. Updating your records at least three times daily—at breakfast, midday, and bedtime—will pay big dividends in your weight-loss journey.

## Challenge #2: Substituting "real food" in place of an entrée

If you want to lose weight quickly, this is not a good idea. Trying to create your own entrée-like servings is not as easy as it sounds. If it were easy, everyone would be doing it and dropping weight—but they're not.

The entrées we recommend are carefully formulated to provide the protein, nutrition, taste, and bulk with the fewest calories possible. They provide automatic portion control—no decisions and no weighing or measuring food.

If you start making your own meals, you may find that your choices will expand day by day. Why not have a small filet mignon steak when you are at a restaurant? More off-diet choices usually lead to more calories, which will slow your weight loss. By sticking with three shakes, two entrées, and five fruits and vegetables daily, you'll lose the weight faster.

## Challenge #3: Falling off the plan

Been there, done that! In the clinic program, patients report going off the plan about one day every two weeks. Since this statistic is based on self-reporting, I believe this is an underestimation and would guess that most people go off the plan at least once weekly. This does not tell us whether they had one small cookie or whether they "grazed" on many different foods the entire day.

The facts show that when people report that they stick with the plan, they lose more weight. Typical on-plan food choices have the following average calorie counts: shakes, 160; entrées, 210; bars, 160; fruits, 50; and vegetables, 40. Fruits and vegetables have only 15 calories per ounce. Most off-plan food choices have far more calories per ounce; some examples include potato chips, 158 calories per ounce; cheese puffs, 160; peanuts, 170; brownies, 120; bacon, 165; and cheese, 108. Thus, any time you go off the plan, you pay a high-calorie price.

If you do go off the plan, however, the important thing is to not let a minor slip become a major plunge. A few peanuts will not hurt as much as mentally giving yourself license to go all-out, since you are already off the plan. If you find yourself having a few peanuts, find some vegetables or fruits, or eat the bar that you have stashed in your purse or briefcase.

Avoiding going off the plan requires planning! Always carry one or two bars in your purse, jacket pocket, briefcase, or car in case you find yourself very hungry.

## Challenge #4: Eating foods that are not on the Simple Diet

This is the most common challenge people on the Simple Diet face. You probably are consuming most of the recommended meal replacements, fruits, and vegetables, but if you are also eating foods not on the diet, try having more foods that *are* on the diet.

Eating more shakes, entrées, fruits, and vegetables is the best way to help you stay on track. Look at the highest levels of intake of meal replacements during your past week on the plan. If, for example, you had four shakes and two entrées, try having five shakes and three entrées one out of the next three days. Many people find that if they increase their number of meal replacements, it keeps them from being hungry and helps them stick with the plan.

Also, if you had six servings of fruits and vegetables as your high for last week, try eating eight servings of fruits and vegetables on a difficult day. The more on-plan foods you include in your day, the less likely you are to eat off-plan foods.

## Challenge #5: Not getting in the minimum number of meal replacements or fruits and vegetables

Maybe you are working hard and using meal replacements, fruits, and vegetables but are having trouble getting in the recommended amount of each. Many of my patients have experienced this challenge. Often, at the same time, other foods are sneaking themselves onto your plate, and you don't know how they got there!

Again, you will find that eating more meal replacements, fruits, and vegetables that are on the Simple Diet will displace the foods that are not on the diet and find their way into your mouth. As with Challenge #4, try to not only meet, but increase your intake of meal replacements, fruits, and vegetables from your best total. Try to increase your intake of shakes by one, entrées by one, and fruits and vegetables by two. Do this in one day out of the next three days and see what happens. We find that this strategy will help you get in your minimum, block intake of those misplaced foods that are appearing mysteriously, and get you back on track to lose weight.

## Challenge #6: Getting hungry between meals and snacks

You are doing a good job of getting in the minimum number of meal replacements, fruits, and vegetables, but you get hungry between times and sometimes develop a little headache. I know the feeling, because I have been there many times.

What do you do? You guessed it: More is better. Instead of having a bar when you are running out of gas, have an entrée.

The average woman in the program can consume seven servings of fruits and vegetables and fourteen (yes, *fourteen!*) meal replacements a day without gaining weight. So if you are getting hungry, try increasing your number of shakes to four or five per day and increase the number of entrées to three or four per day, and you will still probably lose weight. Using more meal replacements helps keep you on the plan and on track to meet your weight-loss goals.

## Challenge #7: Letting your negative self-talk overcome your positive voice

More and more research indicates that we often listen to our negative self-talk ("I can't resist German chocolate cake") instead of being persuaded by our healthy self-talk ("I am in charge of my diet and I can say no to chocolate cake while I am on the Simple Diet"). To overcome negative self-talk, we have to let the positive self-talk be louder. When you catch yourself with a negative thought, replace it with a positive one. Repeat to yourself that you *can* do this—you *can* choose fruit instead of cake at a party, you *can* avoid bringing problem foods into the house, and you *can* get that walk in before going to work. Be your own coach and give yourself a self-talk pep talk. Your positive voice has to be louder than your negative voice to drown it out.

## Challenge #8: Staying on the Simple Diet at a restaurant or social event

Parties and social events present one of the greatest challenges while trying to lose weight. Ideally, you should try to minimize your commitment to these events while you are in the First Phase of the Simple Diet. The fewer restaurants and social events involving meals you go to, the easier your weight loss will be.

However, avoiding these situations and events is not always possible or realistic, so here are some strategies to help you meet this challenge.

- Eat before you go. Have an entrée with vegetables at home ahead of time. Often I make a shake, put it in a thermos mug, and then sip it while my sweet wife is driving to the event. Also, with a hand towel on my lap, I can usually eat an entrée while we are driving without making a mess of the car or myself.
- Suggest a restaurant that has a good selection of vegetable dishes. In most cities I can locate restaurants that feature a vegetable plate on the menu, serve vegetables as side dishes, or have vegetables they serve with entrées. Share with the server that you are on a vegetarian diet. You can start with a green salad—without croutons or cheese—and have a low-calorie dressing on the side. When using the salad dressing, dip the tines of your fork into the dressing and then fork the greens; don't try to pour a little bit onto the salad. Usually you can select several low-calorie vegetables; indicate to the server that you are looking for steamed vegetables instead of fried ones. A baked potato is a good choice, but avoid the butter and sour cream and use salt and pepper for flavor. Many restaurants serve sorbets or sherbets with berries or other fruits; the server can probably find some fruit. A friendly,

"Can you help me with this?" demeanor usually goes a long way to making the server more committed to your special needs.

- Bring your food with you. Many restaurants will heat up an entrée you bring with you. For this special service, I usually call the server over and discreetly display my entrée with a $2 tip on top. I ask servers if they would mind having this heated so I can stay on my special diet. Also, you can order a baked potato and add your own Healthy Choice Hearty Beef Stroganoff to the top (delicious at home or when out). You can empty a shake mix into a water glass and stir with a fork. I once had a shake in a Diet Coke in Disney World, and often bring shakes with me to nice restaurants.

- Make sure you have your three shakes, two entrées, and five fruits and vegetables each day. Getting in all your SEFVs will help you stick with the plan. Even if you do fall off the wagon and eat off the diet, you'll consume fewer calories and have better momentum going into the next day.

## Challenge #9: Staying on the Simple Diet while traveling

If possible, avoid travel away from home by airplane during the First Phase of the diet. But if you do need to travel, plan ahead! Fortunately, you can find shakes and entrées in most U.S. locations. If you are traveling overseas, you should plan to pack your shakes, bars, and shelf-stable entrées and carry on or check this suitcase. Fruits are easier to locate than vegetables in airports and hotels. Plan to purchase entrées that include vegetables—Broccoli & Cheddar Roasted Potatoes (Smart Ones), Italian-style Vegetables and White Chicken (Michelina's), Chili Con Carne with Beans (Weight Watchers), Stuffed Cabbage with Whipped Potatoes (Lean Cuisine)—on your trip so you can get in your entrées and vegetables more readily. Carry enough food in your purse or briefcase to cover your en route time; I always have two bars and two shakes in my briefcase when I fly.

After you check in, find out what the hotel or motel provides and where the nearest market is. You can get in some physical activity by checking out what is available at a nearby convenience store. Recently, near my Washington hotel, a Walgreens had canned fruits and vegetables as well as fresh fruit. The nearest full-service grocery store, the source of a greater variety of choices, was one mile away. Each day I would purchase two frozen entrees and have one for lunch and one for dinner. If you are in a motel, it is likely you will have a microwave in your room or one in the breakfast area that you can use. If you are a hotel guest, it is likely that the hotel restaurant will respect the request of a guest who is ordering salad, vegetables, and/or fruit and heat your entrée. Where there's a will, there's a way.

Eat your Simple Diet foods frequently when you travel. At meetings and conferences, many food choices are usually available, and your best defense against going off the plan is to be fairly full most of the time during the day so the stress of meetings does not prompt you to eat the candy at the table or the pastries at breaks.

During brief breaks, I often dash to my room and have a quick shake or entrée. Many facilities provide microwaves in the rooms. I travel with a small battery-powered stirrer to make shakes. Also, review the tips for restaurant eating outlined in Challenge #8. In a recent three months of travel to ten cities, following these combined strategies saved me 35,000 calories, or about 10 pounds of gained weight.

Recordkeeping is very important when you travel. Since you are out of your routine, it's easy to forget to record your food intake until evening (if not forget it completely!). Whether traveling for pleasure or business, place your records in a prominent place and take them with you. Whether in meetings or out and about, you can record all your meal replacements, fruits, and vegetables.

## Challenge #10: Craving wine or alcohol

Despite the health benefits of red wine, we do not recommend any alcohol intake while in the First Phase of the diet. Alcohol intake adds unnecessary calories and can, for some people, alter their judgment about food choices. Even one drink a day can slow down your weight loss. Plus, they say that willpower dissolves in alcohol!

## Challenge #11: Having trouble reaching 2,000 calories of physical activity weekly

Some people have arthritis or other limitations that make it difficult for them to achieve this physical activity goal. Other participants do not have physical limitations, but have trouble finding the time to work in physical activity. Most of us can do 2,000 calories of physical activity if we could only fit it into our schedule. I know, I've been there! If you have trouble finding a big chunk of time for physical activity, try adding smaller amounts of activity more often throughout the day. Add ten minutes of walking (a half mile) to your schedule. Park farther away from your place of work or from the supermarket and get a little extra walking there. You could walk every aisle of the supermarket. Whatever level of physical activity you are at now, start from there and add in activities. If you can add ten minutes, even in two five-minute sessions, to your daily plan, you will be burning another 75 calories per day, or 500 calories per week.

> "I can enjoy regular physical activity and the positive health effects it provides."

## Challenge #12: You are approaching your goal weight and your weight loss has slowed down

Congratulations, you are almost there! Now is a good time to start practicing the "add volume" key and plan to transition to the Second Phase of the Simple Diet soon. The adding-volume strategy means having more volume but fewer calories.

# Set Yourself Up for Success

If you find your weight loss slowing down, or find yourself having difficulty meeting certain parts of the plan, use the tips in this chapter to help boost your losses and get back on track.

Remember, your best defense against many of the challenges

to weight loss is to eat more—more volume and more on-diet foods, so you will be less tempted to eat off-diet foods. You need to listen to your positive voice that is telling you that you are in charge of your life and you can do this.

Keep your daily progress charts faithfully, and use them to help you identify strengths to capitalize on and weaknesses that need your attention. Acknowledge barriers that could derail your weight-loss progress and step around them. Be proactive, anticipate challenges, and have a plan in place to deal with challenges. If you meet the minimum, stick to the plan, and emphasize volume, you will lose weight.

"I can face weight-loss challenges and know that every effective weight-loss plan starts with a healthy desired weight goal and nonstop determination to reach the goal."

# Health and
# Weight Management:
# Losing Those Last
# Few Pounds and
# Keeping Them Off

*A*ndrew was a carpet store owner with type 2 diabetes. In October of 1990, at age sixty-eight, he was five feet ten inches tall and weighed 255 pounds. He had developed diabetes five years earlier and recently had been placed on forty-two units of insulin daily along with two different pills. He also was taking two blood pressure medicines.

Andrew enrolled in a research study I was conducting and was assigned to the group taking three nutrition shakes daily and eating a 500-calorie evening meal. He began swimming at the YMCA five days per week and walking six days per week. Because his diabetes was well controlled, we reduced his insulin dose to twenty units before he started the diet, and after two weeks, discontinued insulin and all his oral diabetes and hypertension medication.

Andrew lost 48 pounds over twelve weeks. His blood glucose and blood pressure were well controlled with no *medications. After completing the research program, Andrew continued to use meal replacements and began a diet that was high in fiber, low in fat, and rich in whole grains, fruits, and vegetables (the Simple Lifetime Diet I will tell you about later in this chapter and in chapter 12). Andrew lost another 10 pounds over the next three months. He returned to his carpet store with enthusiasm and became an "evangelist" for the weight-loss program!*

*For more than twenty years, Andrew has kept his weight under 200 pounds with the Simple Lifetime Diet and regular physical activity (swimming and walking). He still consumes six to ten servings of fruits and vegetables daily and makes occasional use of shakes and entrées. He is very pleased that he has not had to resume daily insulin injections.*

When you reach your health-promoting weight goal, or are within striking distance, you can transition to the Second Phase, health and weight management. In the Second Phase, you will continue the health-promoting habits you started in the First Phase (the intensive weight-loss phase), plus you'll add a greater variety of foods to your diet. You should plan to continue in the Second Phase for a minimum of six months to practice the skills you have learned in the First Phase. After you've practiced reintegrating healthy low-fat foods during the Second Phase, you can transition to the Simple Lifetime Diet, which is really the same as the Second Phase but with optional use of meal replacements.

You and your doctor can discuss your health- and weight-maintaining weight goal and how much you should lose in the First Phase before transitioning to the Second Phase. Angie (see chapter 3) lost 40 pounds in the First Phase and then went on to lose 20 more pounds in the Second Phase to achieve a non-obese weight. Gloria (see chapter 9) lost 35 pounds in the First Phase and 15 pounds in the Second Phase. Paul (see chapter 6) lost 58 pounds in the First Phase and 9 pounds in the Second Phase. The 100-Pound Club—my patients who lost more than 100 pounds—has over two hundred and fifty members. On average, they lost about two-thirds of their weight (90 pounds) in the First Phase and the remainder (45 pounds) in the Second Phase.

As a general rule, you'll want to lose about 75 percent of the weight you need to lose to achieve a health-maintaining weight in the First Phase and the remaining weight in the Second Phase. If you want to lose less than 40 pounds, you should aim to lose about 80 percent in the First Phase and then transition to the Second Phase. If you want to lose more than 75 pounds, you should lose about two-thirds of it in the First Phase and the remaining one-third in the Second Phase. Thus, if you want to lose 30 pounds, lose 25 pounds in the First Phase; if you need to lose 60 pounds, like Angie, I would recommend you lose 45 pounds in the First Phase.

Just as in the First Phase, there are Six Keys to the Second Phase, health and weight management:

1. Use at least two meal replacements daily (shakes or entrées) in combination with other low-fat foods.
2. Eat at least five servings of fruits and vegetables daily (without added fat or sugar).
3. Add volume and variety (drink a minimum of eight 8-ounce glasses of noncaloric fluids daily

and choose lower-calorie foods, including very lean protein and whole grains).

4. Burn at least 2,000 additional calories in physical activity weekly (about two to three miles, or thirty to forty-five minutes of walking six days weekly).

5. Keep daily summaries of recommended food intake and physical activity.

6. Be accountable to someone (a family member, friend, or your doctor).

You'll notice that all the keys are the same as in the First Phase, except for the first key (use two meal replacements daily instead of five) and the third key (where you are adding volume and variety from many food choices—including fiber-rich whole grains—not just fruits and vegetables). You'll still use two meal replacements daily, but you'll start to choose low-fat, high-nutrition foods in place of the other three meal replacements. You'll gradually reintroduce more food choices, but you'll learn to make those choices wisely. We'll introduce you to our Green Light Calorie Guide to help you with food selection.

# Green Light Calorie Guide

While the Simple Diet does not require you to count calories or grams of fat, obviously you need to recognize health-promoting, low-fat choices compared with heart-attack-risk, high-calorie foods. If you consistently choose high-volume, low-calorie, high-nutrition foods, you will find you are filled up and satisfied on a lower calorie level than if you ate high-fat, low-volume, calorie-dense foods. To help make it easy for you to choose low-calorie foods, I've grouped food choices into four groups.

- **Green Light Foods** contain fewer than 35 calories per ounce and deserve a green light for *Go*—use these foods liberally. For protein-rich foods that are low in calories and high in volume, choose at least two cups of skim milk per day, low-fat cottage cheese, tofu, and egg whites. Most fruits, vegetables, dry cereals, and oatmeal are also green light foods. You can live healthfully getting most of your important nutrients from these foods. If you weigh 180 pounds and wish to lose one pound per week, you can have approximately nine servings from the green category daily.

- **Yellow Light Foods** contain 35 to 70 calories per ounce and can be used in moderation—they get a yellow light for *Caution*, so use these foods judiciously. Protein choices include fish, shellfish, and the white meat from poultry. Very lean beef—including round, flank, sirloin, and tenderloin—grilled or broiled with marble outer layer removed are acceptable. Very lean pork—tenderloin and loin chops—can also be enjoyed. Try to choose your meats from this category, including about three to four ounces of very lean meat or other protein foods daily. Whereas most fruits and vegetables fit in the green light group, avocados, sweet potatoes, potatoes, and beans fall into the yellow category. Whole grain foods such as whole wheat bread also fit in here. If you weigh 180 pounds and wish to lose one pound per week, you can have two servings (like 3 ounces of pork tenderloin) from the yellow category daily.

- **Red Light Foods** contain 70 to 110 calories per ounce. The red light demands a full *Stop* to give this choice all due consideration. These foods should be monitored carefully. Red light foods include most cuts of red meat, fried vegetables, muffins, bagels, cakes, cookies, and most pies. As a general rule, if you are heavier than you want to be, you should avoid these foods.

- **Flashing-Red-Alert Foods** are foods that you should try to avoid, with the possible exception of nuts and olive oil. Imagine that these foods come with a strobing red light and a blaring siren: *Danger*. This category includes processed meats such as sausage and bologna, most "crinkly bag" snacks such as chips and crackers, and most sweets and desserts. If you are trying to lose weight, you should pretend that you have a severe allergy to the red-alert foods. One friend with a chocolate allergy cannot even sit at the table next to someone eating chocolate—and neither should you! Nuts are high in nutrition values but also pack in about 160 calories per ounce—more than five times the calories per ounce than green light foods. However, because of their health benefits, persons already at a healthy body weight could include one ounce (about ¼ cup) of almonds, walnuts, pistachios, or other nuts daily. Very modest amounts of olive oil daily—one to two teaspoons—may also have beneficial effects on heart health for persons already at a healthy body weight.

The calorie values used in the Green Light Calorie Guide are based on average values. The foods you eat may vary slightly from this guide based on the brand you choose or how you prepare the food. You can divide the calorie values given for the food by the number of ounces per serving to get calories per ounce. If serving size is given in grams, divide the grams by 28 to estimate ounces. Compare calories per ounce to the calorie values given in the top row to determine the color category for the food.

## GREEN LIGHT CALORIE GUIDE

| FOOD | GREEN <br> < 35 CALORIES/ OZ. (USE LIBERALLY) | YELLOW <br> 35–70 CALORIES/ OZ. (USE JUDI- CIOUSLY) | RED <br> 70–110 CALORIES/ OZ. (AVOID OR USE SPARINGLY) | RED ALERT <br> >110 CALORIES/ OZ. (AVOID) |
|---|---|---|---|---|
| **Protein** <br> (Include at least 2 servings of non-fat milk or soy milk and three to four ounces of very lean meat or other protein foods daily) | Non-fat milk, regular or soy <br><br> Non-fat yogurt, regular or soy <br><br> Cottage cheese, low-fat <br><br> Tofu <br><br> Egg whites <br><br> Egg substitutes | Fish <br><br> Shell fish <br><br> Turkey breast w/o skin <br><br> Chicken breast w/o skin <br><br> Beef, very lean <br><br> Pork, very lean <br><br> Vegetarian burger <br><br> Cottage cheese | Beef, lean <br><br> Pork, lean <br><br> Cheese, low-fat and non-fat | Pork sausage <br><br> Fried foods <br><br> Hot dogs <br><br> Pizza <br><br> Bacon <br><br> Cheese, regular |
| **Fruits and Vegetables** <br> (Include at least five servings of fruits and vegetables daily; see appendices 10.2 and 10.3 for serving sizes) | Fruits, almost all <br><br> Vegetables, almost all <br><br> Vegetable soup | Avocados <br><br> Edamame <br><br> Dried beans and peas <br><br> Potatoes <br><br> Sweet potato | Vegetables, fried | French fries <br><br> Potato chips <br><br> Tortilla chips |

| FOOD | GREEN<br><br>< 35 CALORIES/ OZ.<br>(USE LIBERALLY) | YELLOW<br><br>35–70 CALORIES/ OZ. (USE JUDI-CIOUSLY) | RED<br><br>70–110 CALORIES/ OZ.<br>(AVOID OR USE SPARINGLY) | RED ALERT<br><br>>110 CALORIES/ OZ.<br>(AVOID) |
|---|---|---|---|---|
| **Cereals and Grains**<br>(Include three whole grains daily) | Oatmeal<br>Cereal, high-fiber, dry, most | Pancakes<br>Whole-wheat bread<br>English muffins<br>Pasta, whole-wheat<br>Pasta<br>Rice, white and brown | Bagels<br>Bread, white<br>Muffins<br>Popcorn, plain, air-popped | Crackers<br>Granola cereals, most |
| **Fats and Sweets** | Salad dressing, low-calorie<br>Butter buds<br>Condiments such as ketchup, mustard, and many others<br>Low-calorie jelly and jam<br>Low-calorie syrup<br>Artificial sweeteners | | Angel food cake<br>Cookies<br>Fruit pies<br>Yellow cake | Cake, most<br>Candy<br>Candy bars<br>Nuts, all<br>Margarine<br>Butter<br>Oils |

You don't need to count calories as you introduce new foods, but just decide into which category the food fits, then pick generously from green light choices, moderately from yellow light choices, and very sparingly from red light choices. When you load your plate with low-fat, low-calorie, high-volume foods, your diet will naturally be low in calories without having to keep track of them. If you find you are struggling to keep your weight loss off, choose more green light foods. If you are physically active and keeping your weight off easily, you will have more flexibility to choose foods from yellow and red categories. For individuals who want more detailed guidance, Appendix 10.1 gives an expanded version of the Green Light Calorie Guide with suggested servings sizes for green, yellow, and red foods. Appendix 10.1 also gives Nutrition Quality Scores to indicate those foods that provide the highest quality of nutrition per serving.[41] Not surprisingly, virtually all of the excellent and very good quality scores are given to foods in the green zone. As a further guide to food choices, appendices 10.2 and 10.3 give suggestions for the number of servings of foods in the various zones to aim for for persons at different weights who are either desiring to lose more weight or are content to maintain their current weights.

# Making the Transition from the First Phase to the Second Phase of the Simple Diet

When entering the Second Phase, the health and weight management phase, you are really transitioning from an intensive diet to lose weight to a healthy low-fat, high-fiber diet that everyone can and should follow for life, even if they don't need to lose weight. We recommend that you remain in the Second Phase of the Simple Diet for at least six months to sustain the healthy nutrition, physical activity, and monitoring habits you have developed in the First Phase.

After you have followed the Second Phase for at least six months, you can transition to the Simple Lifetime Diet, a healthy way for everyone to eat for life. The Simple Lifetime Diet is really the same as the Second Phase except meal replacements are optional. It is made up of mostly green light foods with a smattering of yellow light foods. In the latest dietary advice to all Americans, the U.S. Department of Agriculture recommends your plate be over three-fourths full of vegetables, fruits, and whole grains—exactly what the Simple Lifetime Diet recommends (www.choosemyplate.gov).

Some people who really struggle with weight stay in the Second Phase for life, following a healthy low-fat diet, but needing the simple no-decision aspect of calorie control that meal replacements provide for certain meals or certain days of the week. And if they hit a rough spot or regain some pounds, they go back to using more meal replacements, as in the First Phase, to bring them back on track. Below is a sample three-day menu for the Second Phase of the Simple Diet. This diet provides about 1,400 calories per day and is designed to empower a person weighing about 180 pounds to continue losing approximately one pound per week.

## SAMPLE THREE-DAY MENU FOR SECOND PHASE

| MEAL | DAY 1 | DAY 2 | DAY 3 |
|---|---|---|---|
| **Breakfast** | ½ cup cooked oatmeal with 8 oz. skim milk, 1 cup blackberries and blueberries | 1 cup Cheerios with 1 cup skim milk, grapefruit half | ¾ cup Raisin Bran with 1 cup skim milk, 1 cup cantaloupe |
| **Snack** | 1 cup carrots, celery, cherry tomatoes, and red pepper strips with 1 tbsp. no-fat ranch dressing | 2 cups coffee, decaf coffee, or tea with ¼ cup skim milk, Splenda to taste | Strawberry shake (Special K) |
| **Lunch** | 3 cups tossed green salad with cherry tomatoes and 3 oz. chicken breast strips, low-fat salad dressing, whole wheat roll, 1 pear | Small garden salad with low-fat dressing, 6-inch Subway Veggie Delite sandwich, 1 banana | Mixed green salad with low-calorie dressing, Herb Roasted Chicken (Lean Cuisine), 1 cup mixed steamed vegetables, ½ cup mandarin oranges |

| MEAL | DAY 1 | DAY 2 | DAY 3 |
|---|---|---|---|
| **Snack** | Vanilla Pleasure shake mix (Revival Soy) blended with ½ cup strawberries | French Vanilla shake (Slim-Rite) | 1 cup carrots, celery, cherry tomatoes, and red pepper strips with 1 tbsp. no-fat ranch dressing |
| **Dinner** | 3 cups spinach salad with low-calorie dressing, Teriyaki Chicken & Vegetables (Smart Ones), 1 cup green beans, 1 cup mixed fresh fruit medley | Lettuce and tomato salad with low-fat dressing, 3 oz. grilled pork tenderloin, 1 cup mashed potatoes, 1 cup green beans, whole wheat roll, 1 peach | Spinach salad with low-calorie dressing, 3 oz. broiled salmon, ½ cup garlic mashed potatoes, 1 cup steamed broccoli, 1 cup mixed fruit salad |
| **Snack** | 1 cup mixed fruit salad | 1 orange | Whole wheat toast with 1 tbsp. Crofter's Just Fruit strawberry spread |

In the Second Phase, you will continue enjoying an enormous range of fruits and vegetables. In addition, you will include three to four ounces of very lean protein, two cups of skim milk, and three servings of whole grains.

*Randy was forty-seven years old when he had his heart attack in 1967. He was too obese for heart surgery, and his cardiologist referred him to me to lose weight so he could have coronary artery bypass surgery. Weighing in at 301 pounds and standing slightly under six feet tall, Randy was eager to lose 100 pounds. This construction company owner earnestly began the very-low-calorie diet we were using in the clinic program and started walking two miles daily three weeks after his heart attack. He lost 50 pounds in eight weeks and dropped another 55 pounds in eleven more weeks in the First*

*Phase. He transitioned to the Second Phase to complete his weight loss and "graduated" at a weight of 177 pounds. I counseled him on the Simple Lifetime Diet, and he came in to see me every two to three months.*

*Randy was one of the first people to begin the Simple Lifetime Diet. For twenty-two years, he consumed the high-fiber, low-fat diet with three servings of whole grains and at least eight servings of fruits and vegetables daily. He walked three to four miles daily and maintained a weight between 185 and 210 pounds most of the time. When his weight crept up over 210 pounds, he came back to the program and took a six-week refresher course using meal replacements. He used two or more shakes or entrées on most days for more than twenty years, never required heart surgery, and passed a number of heart stress tests with flying colors.*

We recommend that you strictly follow the Second Phase key guidelines for a minimum of six months as Randy did. This structure lets you reenter the world of many food choices gradually, while still keeping records and being accountable, reinforcing habits that will serve you all your life. During this phase you will learn how to manage episodes of overeating by quickly returning to meal replacements, fruits, and vegetables, and how to manage your food intake during holidays, special events, and travel. When you have developed a rhythm and are managing your health-promoting weight for at least six months, then the use of meal replacements becomes optional. However, many of my patients, like Randy, have used shakes and entrées as part of their health-promoting diets for many years.

"I can maintain my health-promoting weight using two meal replacements, fruits, vegetables, and the Green Light Calorie Guide."

## The Simple Lifetime Diet for Health and Weight Management

We have been developing the Simple Lifetime Diet for more than thirty-five years to preserve health and reverse disease processes such as diabetes and heart disease. On the Simple Lifetime Diet, you'll be eating essentially how you ate in the Second Phase, except meal replacements are optional. You'll still eat lots of high-volume vegetables, fruits, and whole grains and choose mostly foods from the green zone of the Green Light Calorie Guide.

Thousands of our patients have successfully used this diet for long-term health and weight management, including Andrew and Randy. In chapter 12, I'll provide more specific details on the Simple Lifetime Diet and guide you in other healthful behaviors to enhance your weight and health management.

# Keep the Weight Off for Good

You might wonder whether the effort of losing weight is worth it. Maybe you're afraid you'll gain the weight right back when you start making all your own food choices. We've all heard stories or even personally experienced losing 10 to 15 pounds only to regain 15 to 20. Well, I have good news for you! Careful studies show that most people who lose more than 20 pounds keep most of the weight off over the long term. My own research shows that most individuals who lose more than 20 pounds keep more than 10 pounds off for five years or longer.[42] Further, people who have lost more than 100 pounds on the program keep an average of 65 pounds off for five years.[43]

Keeping the weight off, however, doesn't just happen, and it's not always easy. Two major factors contribute to this challenge. First, changing habits that have been established over ten, twenty, or thirty years or more is *not* a snap. I know—I was overweight for many years. Although I was active and ate healthfully, I had to make changes in my habits to achieve and maintain a health-promoting weight. On the positive side, I increased my walking, started fitness activities, and ate more fruits and vegetables—at least eight servings per day. On the negative side, I gave up desserts almost completely and minimized my intake of high-fat animal products.

Second, when we lose a moderate to large amount of weight—more than 30 pounds—our metabolism slows down, so we require fewer calories per pound to maintain our current weight than we did before we lost the weight. So let's face the fact that to succeed at keeping pounds off for life, we need to replace old bad habits with new healthy ones.

# Habits of Those
# Who've Kept the Weight Off

The National Weight Control Registry was established by Dr. Rena Wing and Dr. James Hill in 1993. This registry includes detailed information on successful dieters who have lost more than 30 pounds and have kept off more than 30 pounds for at least one year. Over the last eighteen years, Wing, Hill, and their associates have reported weight and behavior data for over five thousand individuals and have published more than twenty-five research papers on factors related to keeping weight off. Three major habits vital to maintaining a healthy lifetime weight stand out.

- Obtain regular physical activity.
- Eat generous amounts of fruits and vegetables.
- Systematically eat a low-fat diet.

To provide a little more detail, researchers have confirmed the benefits of walking more than sixty minutes (three miles) daily; high levels of fruit and vegetable intake; high fiber intake from fruits, vegetables, and whole grains; and low fat intakes. Several studies suggest that fat intake should be less than 25 percent of total calorie intake. The National Weight Control Registry data indicate that people who are successful at weight maintenance weigh themselves frequently and eat regular meals in addition to eating a low-calorie, low-fat diet and achieving a high level of physical activity. Further, 80 percent of people who were successfully keeping the weight off ate breakfast. Regular self-monitoring of weight, spending less time watching television (two-thirds of people who keep their weight off watch less than ten hours per week), and less consumption of fast food also contribute to keeping the weight off.

The consistency of diet regimen is also important: Those who keep to their commitment to maintaining their healthy diet on weekends and holidays as well as on ordinary days have significantly better weight maintenance results than those who only focus on a consistent diet during weekdays. Limiting choices and eating only a small variety of high-fat foods is also associated with keeping the weight off. For example, some people make all low-fat food choices, except they will use a small amount of margarine or olive oil to top certain foods. Maintaining a relationship with a weight-loss group, counselor, or support system is also associated with keeping weight off.

## Twelve Key Practices to Stay at Your Health-Promoting Weight for Life

Let's talk turkey (a good protein choice in your weight management phase!) about the most important features of your health and weight management plan. These practices apply to the Second Phase and also to the Simple Lifetime Diet for health and weight management. While there are numerous health-promoting practices you are likely to hear or read about and may feel you'll want to try as overall fit living becomes your permanent lifestyle, we have summarized here what we consider the twelve most important practices to maintaining your health-promoting weight for life.

## 1. Keep Up the Physical Activity.

Since your metabolism slows down after your weight loss, you'll need to pick up the physical activity to burn extra calories. We recommend you initially establish a habit of walking or doing equivalent activities for forty-five minutes daily, six days per week. This time recommendation is a general guideline and may need to be tweaked to be optimal for you. If it's difficult for you to devote a single forty-five-minute block of time to walking, it is just as effective to take three fifteen-minute walks.

Regular physical activity is reported by more than 87 percent of participants in the National Weight Control Registry, with 75 percent reporting more than 1,000 calories per week (walking about ten miles), and 54 percent expending more than 2,000 calories per week (walking about twenty miles).

The most common physical activities for successful dieters are walking (72 percent), resistance training (29 percent), cycling (18 percent), aerobics (16 percent), cardio machines (15 percent), running (14 percent), floor conditioning (10 percent), and swimming (5 percent). The weight-loss literature suggests that the total calories expended in physical activity rather than the type of physical activity (low- versus high-intensity) is the most important attribute for successful weight maintenance.

## 2. Eat a Low-Fat Diet.

Becoming a "fat detective"—an expert in discovering the fat content of everything you eat—is vital to your success. High intakes of fat, especially animal fat from meat and dairy products, are a major health hazard. In addition to increasing risk for heart attack, stroke, diabetes, and breast cancers, high fat intake is your number-one enemy in keeping the weight off. Your goal is to eat a low-fat, low-calorie diet day in and day out. The general recommendation is to eat a diet containing less than 25 percent of calories from fat. This means that almost all of your food choices will have less than 3 grams of fat per 100 calories. Choosing about 80 percent of your foods from the green calorie zone will help you meet this goal. See appendices 10.2 and 10.3 for more specific guides to green and yellow zone food selections.

### 3. Eat Plenty of Fruits and Vegetables.

As a fat detective, you'll see that eating plenty of plain fruits and vegetables is a no-brainer. All fresh, frozen, and canned vegetables are good low-fat choices—even baked potatoes. These foods are filling and full of fiber. I recommend a minimum of five servings every day, but personally often enjoy ten per day. Avoid canned fruit and vegetables that have added sugar or high-fructose corn syrup and tons of sodium. You can rinse these foods thoroughly with cold water to get rid of sugar and salt, but if you have the option of fresh or even frozen, is it really worth the hassle?

"I can continue to consume at least five servings of fruits and vegetables daily because of their broad health and weight management benefits."

## 4. Use Meal Replacements Strategically.

During the Second Phase, you will use two meal replacements daily. This will help you stay on track as you gradually add other foods back into your diet. I recommend at least one entrée and one shake daily. As you transition out of the Second Phase to the Simple Lifetime Diet, you many decide to forgo meal replacements entirely, although I personally have used one to three meal replacements daily for more than twenty years to maintain a health-promoting body weight. Research indicates that individuals who use meal replacements regularly as part of their weight management efforts gain 25 fewer pounds over ten years than people who do not use meal replacements.[44]

Meal replacements are especially useful when traveling to help keep my weight in check. Meal replacements will also help you if you slip a little. Even the healthiest eaters may overindulge occasionally and can add a few pounds after holidays, vacations, etc. Our research and studies by many other obesity investigators show that daily use of meal replacements—shakes or entrées—after a little weight gain is a very effective tool to help you get the weight back off.

## 5. Always Eat Breakfast.

Research studies time after time show that keeping the weight off is easier when individuals enjoy a hearty breakfast. Try starting your day out with a high-volume breakfast, such as a high-fiber cereal and fruit. Oatmeal with fruit is one of the very best breakfast choices.

## 6. Weigh Yourself Regularly.

People who are successful at keeping the weight off for life are constantly monitoring their weight. Regular self-monitoring of your weight allows you to see right away when your eating and exercise habits are not working and lets you do something about it early on—before much damage has been done. The National Weight Control Registry data show that 36 percent of individuals who have kept weight off successfully weigh themselves daily, and 79 percent weigh themselves weekly. Individuals who weigh themselves frequently eat less fat and gain less weight than individuals who weigh themselves less frequently.

## 7. Keep Track of Your Weight and Other Activities.

Many people who successfully keep weight off continue to monitor not only their weight, but also other health habits, keeping track in a notebook or computer program. Keeping at least rough track of your physical activity and even foods eaten will help you assess if your habits are working for you. And remember, individuals who eat a consistent low-fat diet on weekends and holidays maintain their weight better than people who focus on a consistent diet on weekdays but give themselves some leeway on weekends and holidays. Keeping track every day will help you stay on track every day.

## 8. Limit Television Watching.

Two-thirds of successful weight maintainers watch less than ten hours of television weekly, whereas some couch potatoes can watch ten hours of television on a weekend day. In addition to doing yourself a favor, parents who limit television themselves will be setting a good example for their kids. Research clearly shows that children who watch the most television are heavier than children who watch the least television weekly.

## 9. Strictly Limit Fast Food.

Successful weight maintainers only rarely patronize fast-food restaurants. Many fast foods are fat- and calorie-laden, and you usually have to hunt pretty hard to find the fresh fruits and vegetables at fast-food restaurants.

## 10. Establish Healthy Lifetime Eating Habits and Follow Them Conscientiously.

Successful weight maintainers have developed new eating habits that they follow regularly. They eat breakfast to start their day with fruit and fiber. They plan their days so they do not encounter surprises for which they are not prepared. They often have shakes, entrées, or bars stashed in strategic places so they always have healthy choices. They stock their kitchen with healthy food choices such as fruits, vegetables, whole grains, and low-fat protein sources so they can prepare a meal without running to the grocery store. They tend to eat the same way on weekends and holidays as they do during the week. This takes planning and some work, but the results are surely worth it.

## 11. Keep Moving.

While I have focused on physical activity during weight loss and maintenance, your real health goal is *physical fitness*. Physical fitness involves cardiovascular and aerobic exercises like brisk walking, strength training with the use of free weights or machines, and stretching. Our recommendation is that you enroll in a local YMCA, gym, or fitness club and get an evaluation and individualized program. Optimally, going to the gym three times weekly and doing strength training for about forty-five to sixty minutes would be a good goal. The stretching exercises could be accomplished in a few minutes each day after your daily aerobic activity.

You don't have to start running marathons, but consistent long-term physical fitness will not only help you maintain your weight loss, it will also have an incredibly positive impact on your overall health.

## 12. Maintain a Positive, Can-Do Attitude.

Having a positive, can-do attitude and maintaining confidence in yourself and your ability to develop and sustain health-promoting habits are very important in health management. Practice your affirming self-talk until it becomes second nature and displaces negative self-talk. Replace "I can't follow my diet at a buffet" with "I can choose plenty of fresh vegetables and fruits from the salad bar, maybe add a little fish, and bring a shake or bar in the car if needed." Positive self-talk works. It will give you the confidence to practice health-promoting behaviors consistently.

> "I can maintain affirming self-talk and not accept negative, demeaning self-talk."

# What about Eating Out?

Many restaurants are happy to cater to special requests, especially for a polite customer who is likely to leave a generous tip. Ask that your vegetables be steamed or boiled rather than sautéed in oil. Fish or poultry can usually be prepared plain (poached, grilled, roasted, or steamed) with sauces served on the side, and a fresh fruit cup substituted for something chosen from the usual "dangerous dessert" list. If you are going to the restaurant at a busy time, call ahead to ask if they can accommodate your requests, and if not, choose a different restaurant.

Be cautious of even entering a fast-food restaurant, and stay out of the drive-thru lane. A typical fast-food meal at McDonald's, Pizza Hut, or KFC can contain in excess of 1,000 calories. *Do you hear the siren?* Even one of these fast-food meals per week can set you back. If you avoid the high-fat dressing, cheese, and croutons, though, you can often get a dinner salad at many fast-food restaurants. And some fast-food chains also carry a few items from the yellow category: plain baked potatoes or corn on the cob (though you'll probably have to specially request that they not add margarine or butter to the corn).

Here are some more suggestions for low-calorie eating out:

- Ask for water with extra lemons and make your own lemonade.
- Ask for raw veggies in place of bread.
- Request steamed or boiled vegetables rather than fried vegetables or vegetables in sauces.
- With salads, ask for a non-fat dressing or plain vinegar, or ask for dressing served on the side and only dip your fork in it as you eat the salad.

- Ask the server to remove the bread or chip basket from the table.
- Explain your diet needs to your server, and ask them to ask the chef how dishes are prepared if needed.
- Wines having about 20 calories per ounce, or 80 to 100 calories for a glass, are good choices compared with liquors having about 65 to 85 calories per ounce. Remember that willpower dissolves in alcohol!

Most restaurants, even those famous for their high-fat items, have fruit and vegetable choices. Recently, after my sister-in-law's retirement reception, we all went out to dinner. Bob Evans would not have been my first choice, but that is what the family found convenient. I had a tossed salad, removed the croutons, and used about a teaspoon of low-calorie dressing. Then I had steamed broccoli and a baked potato with about a teaspoon of sour cream. For dessert I had a fruit cup with grapes, pineapple, and melon. I had a nutrition bar in the car and had a meal replacement entrée when we got home.

# Your Long-Term Success

By the time you get to this point, I'm pretty sure you must be pleased with your success in weight loss and are eager to continue that success as you transition from the Second Phase to the Simple Lifetime Diet. You have developed a rhythm of getting physical activity into your schedule, and you recognize the contribution this makes to your weight management, mood, and general quality of life. On the Simple Diet, you have learned that you can survive without hamburgers, French fries, bacon, sausage, well-marbled steak, and ice cream (all in the red light category). For long-term success, you will have to allow yourself these items only rarely. By now you have determined which fruits and vegetables you enjoy, how to prepare them in tasty dishes, and how they complement other foods. Continue these behaviors. You have likely lost much weight and gained something invaluable—health! Keep up the good work!

"I can make healthy nutrition choices and exercise regularly to maintain my health because I know weight management is vital for health management."

# Bariatric Surgery: It's Really Risky— and the Last Resort

Harriet was a forty-seven-year-old disabled high school math teacher who came to see me about her persistent weight problem after gastric bypass surgery. This unfortunate lady had been obese since high school and had developed sleep apnea requiring the use of a CPAP machine. At five feet four inches, she had weighed 251 pounds prior to gastric bypass surgery five months earlier. Her sister described her as a gregarious, very bright woman with countless friends before her surgery.

Immediately after surgery they were unable to wake her up, and the neurologist concluded that her brain had not received adequate oxygen during the operation. The diagnosis was postoperative cognitive dysfunction. After being in a coma for more than one month, she had awakened. After two months in a rehab facility, this single lady had been taken home by her sister and was gradually *beginning to be more independent. Although she had no trouble walking, she had lost cognitive function similarly to a person with moderately severe Alzheimer's disease. She could not drive and got lost very easily. She still was very personable, but struggled to find words when talking to me.*

*This formerly dynamic teacher who had won many teaching awards obviously could not resume teaching. She was able to eat fairly normally—unusual after this operation—and had lost only 23 pounds after surgery. She and her sister wanted my guidance on what she could do to lose further weight. We assessed her vitamin and mineral status and started on an intensive regimen of supplemental vitamins and minerals. The dietitian and I counseled them on choosing low-fat foods and consuming fairly high amounts of fruits and vegetables.*

Hundreds of people have sought my advice about having some sort of bariatric or stomach surgery for weight loss. More than 90 percent of the time, I have encouraged them to commit to an intensive weight-loss program using lifestyle measures instead. In my opinion, a lifestyle weight-loss program like the Simple Diet is both safer and more effective. Yes, *more* effective, over both the short term and the long term. Our lifestyle intervention empowers 20 percent of individuals with severe obesity who enter the program to lose more than 100 pounds.

# The Good, the Bad, and the Extremely Ugly

Bariatric surgery is *good* news for people who have tried very hard to achieve and maintain a health-promoting weight and have not been successful. The average individual who has gastric bypass surgery loses 85 pounds in one year and is down 69 pounds after six years.[45] As a weight-loss intervention, bariatric surgery has dramatic effects on diabetes, usually reversing type 2 diabetes, and individuals who have had gastric bypass surgery have increased survival compared with equally obese persons who do not lose the weight. These benefits have been attributed to achieving a more health-protective weight and would likely be seen in patients who have long-term success with any weight-loss program.

The *bad* news is that the short-term risk of death after gastric bypass surgery averages about 1 percent (one in one hundred) within one month and 1.6 percent (one in sixty-three) within one year.[46,47] The complication rate averages about 40 percent.[48] Most people will have gastrointestinal problems for the rest of their lives. Serious nutritional deficiencies with severe neuropathy, osteoporosis, decreased cognitive function (Alzheimer's-type symptoms), emotional problems, and anemia are common. Harriet is an example of a very bad outcome from bariatric surgery.

The *extremely ugly* part is that bariatric surgery is heavily marketed and is an important profit center for some hospitals and medical groups. About 220,000 American adolescents and adults have bariatric surgery annually, at costs exceeding $6 billion. Now some surgeons are pushing to perform bariatric surgery for persons with mild obesity!

Some obese individuals are vulnerable to the lure of a quick and easy fix for their weight problem. Procedures that have not stood the test of time—experimental procedures such as gastric sleeves—are being promoted, often to non-obese individuals and adolescents.

# History of Bariatric Surgery

Although it's never been the epidemic we are seeing today, obesity is a problem that has long been with us. For more than fifty years, academic surgeons at university medical schools have attempted to develop safe and effective gastrointestinal operations to facilitate weight loss.

The first effective and relatively safe surgical procedure was vertical banded gastroplasty, developed in 1966. It is performed much less frequently today because of less favorable long-term weight loss and side effects including gastroesophageal reflux disease (stomach acid reflux into the esophagus) and solid food intolerance.

Gastric bypass surgery was first reported in 1967, and the Roux-en-Y gastric bypass (RYGB) developed subsequently. When laparoscopic procedures became available, the RYGB became the most effective bariatric procedure.

In 2001, the Food and Drug Administration approved the LAP-BAND device and procedure for bariatric surgery. Laparoscopic adjustable gastric banding (LAGB) surgery has gained extreme popularity because it can be done quickly and only requires hospitalization for one night if there are no complications.

Entrepreneurial surgeons have developed other approaches, such as the mini gastric bypass. Unlike prescription drugs and devices such as the LAP-BAND, new surgical procedures do not have to obtain formal approval and depend on the standards of the local community or hospital. Unfortunately, a wide variety of newer procedures are now being promoted without reliable information on their safety or effectiveness.

One of the major problems with bariatric surgical procedures is the lack of accurate information about mortality, complications, and long-term weight loss. Less than one-third of deaths from bariatric procedures occur in the hospital, so hospital mortality grossly underestimates actual death rates related to the procedure. Statewide studies covering longer periods of time probably also underestimate death rates, though to a lesser degree, because individuals may have moved out of state. No good prospective studies in the United States systematically track patients after surgery or have follow-up information on almost 100 percent of participants. Even standardized data collection systems are very restrictive in the type of data collected, and thus provide underestimates of complications. In providing mortality estimates, I have relied on reports using statewide or national data rather than those from individual case series.

Estimating rates of complications from surgical procedures is difficult because this information is not collected systematically unless it is part of a study for regulatory approval, such as the LAP-BAND study or the National Surgical Quality Improvement Program. I have participated in hundreds of clinical trials related to drugs or supplements where we systematically collected information on side effects. Our research coordinators were trained to do this, monitors reviewed our records regularly, and we had to be prepared for FDA audits. This type of detailed information is not available for bariatric surgical procedures, and even reports from the Swedish Obesity Study—a long-term follow-up of individuals who have had bariatric surgery in Sweden—provide limited information about side effects or surgical mortality.[49] After a detailed review of over eighty articles, I have made estimates about the types and rates of complications. These references are available at andersonsimplediet.com.

# Types of Bariatric Procedures

There are three main types of bariatric surgery: Roux-en-Y gastric bypass (RYGB), laparoscopic adjustable gastric banding (LAGB), and the gastric sleeve. LAGB is very popular, quick and easy for the surgeon and patient, but in my opinion is less effective and the long-term success rates are not well documented. Various forms of gastric sleeve operations are emerging, but the safety and efficacy of these experimental procedures are not documented.

RYGB surgery now is usually done laparoscopically, which eliminates a large scar and hastens recovery. This procedure involves creating a small stomach pouch that is divided from the rest of the stomach and connected to a segment of the small intestine. Food thus bypasses the stomach and enters the small intestine below the secretions coming from the gallbladder and pancreas. The small pouch, unlike a large-volume stomach, limits the amount of food that can be consumed at one time, and the bypass of the gallbladder and pancreas decreases the absorption of some of the calories and nutrients. The risks include some serious surgical complications, for example, pulmonary embolism (a blood clot that goes to the lungs), intestinal leak, infections, bleeding, and staple line failure. Long-term problems include a host of gastrointestinal problems, nutritional deficiencies, and neurological and psychiatric problems. Complications notwithstanding, this is the procedure that I steer people toward when very occasionally I do recommend bariatric surgery.

LAGB can be done quickly and usually requires only one night in the hospital unless there are complications. An adjustable silicone band is placed around the upper part of the stomach to create a small pouch and restricted outlet. Saline (sterile salt water) can be injected into or removed from the band to change the diameter of the outlet. The band can be removed if there are problems, and it needs to be replaced periodically. Mortality from this procedure is only 20 to 30 percent of that for RYGB, but weight loss appears to be about one-third less than RYGB. However, complication rates and rehospitalization rates are higher for LAGB than for RYGB.

The gastric sleeve operation is done by placing a large tube through the mouth and down into the duodenum. Laparoscopically, the stomach is stapled around the tube in such a way that when the tube is withdrawn there is a narrow sleeve through which food passes from the esophagus to the duodenum. The stomach outside the sleeve is usually removed, leaving a rather narrow tube where the high-capacity stomach once was. In my view, this is an experimental procedure, and the safety and efficacy for even one year have not been documented. Unfortunately, as I've mentioned, unlike approval of drugs by the FDA, surgical procedures do not require a formal approval, so a surgeon can invent a new procedure and simply start doing it.

# Deaths from Bariatric Surgery

Deaths from surgery are often categorized in three ways: in the hospital, within thirty days of surgery, and within one year after surgery. After gastric bypass surgery, the death rates are approximately one in two hundred in the hospital. Within thirty days, about one in one hundred die, and within the year, one in sixty-three die. Most bariatric surgeons will tell you that rates are much lower than these.

The most common complications leading to death after gastric bypass surgery are leakage from one of the new intestinal connections that have been made, a pulmonary embolism, heart problems, infections, and internal bleeding.

After LAGB surgery, the rates of death are much lower. In the hospital, deaths are about one in 1,000; the thirty-day rate is about one in 333; and the one-year rate is about one in 200. At least one factor in these lower rates is that the majority of LAGB patients are young women who are barely 100 pounds overweight.

*Laura, a thirty-eight-year-old teacher, weighed 235 pounds at five feet six inches and qualified to have an LAGB procedure. Over the next year she lost 55 pounds, and now her weight has stabilized at 170 pounds. She vomits frequently due to misgauging the limits of her stomach's reduced capacity and cannot enjoy holidays or special events because her food choices and amounts are severely restricted. Prior to choosing to undergo this procedure, Laura had not attempted a serious-minded effort at weight loss. Many of my patients who had similar weight problems have achieved similar weight losses and can still enjoy holidays and special events.*

Two major factors affect mortality rates: the medical risks of the patient and the experience of the surgeon and supporting team. A person with low medical risks has a risk for death in the hospital after gastric bypass surgery of 0.2 percent (one in five hundred), and a person with moderate risk of 1.1 percent (one in ninety-one). The individual with sleep apnea, diabetes, heart disease, or a combination of medical risks is at high risk, and the death rate in the hospital is about 2.4 percent (one in forty-two).

If you are seriously considering bariatric surgery, you should choose the most experienced surgeon and hospital support team that you can. The risk for death from bariatric surgery (including RYGB and LAGB) for highly experienced groups is 0.2 percent (one in five hundred), for moderately experienced groups is 0.4 percent (one in 250), and for less experienced groups 1.1 percent (one in ninety-one). Ideally, the hospital has been supporting bariatric surgery for more than five years and the surgeon has done over five hundred bariatric procedures.

# Complications after Gastric Bypass Surgery

The complications rate after gastric bypass surgery approaches 40 percent in the first year. For about 20 percent of patients, these complications require another hospitalization, and for about 8 percent of patients, a second operation. These rates are high because gastric bypass surgery requires major rearranging of the anatomy of the stomach and small intestine. This procedure affects stomach and intestinal functions—functions we use many times daily—and creates, in fact, forms of partial gastrointestinal obstruction.

The most common problems encountered in the hospital are pulmonary embolism, pneumonia, blood clots in the legs or large veins of the abdomen, infections, intestinal bleeding, and heart problems. All patients have some gastrointestinal problems that often include vomiting, acid reflux, and dumping syndrome (a rapid emptying of food from the tiny stomach pouch into the small intestine). The dumping syndrome can cause nausea, vomiting, abdominal cramping, bloating, diarrhea, dizziness, fatigue, and rapid heart rates.

In the month after surgery, gastrointestinal symptoms continue in most people. These include nausea, vomiting, diarrhea, and the dumping syndrome. Over time, these symptoms diminish as patients develop an eating pattern and ideally find food choices that allow them to tolerate eating and obtain adequate nutrition. The most troublesome symptoms that are seen are leaking from some of the intestinal connections, experienced by 10.6 percent of all patients; narrowing of the opening between the stomach and intestine, 8 percent of patients; ulcers in the small intestine, 3 percent; and intestinal bleeding, 1.5 percent. During this period, nutrition problems such as low protein levels in the blood, anemia, and other signs of nutritional deficiency may develop.

Over the year following surgery, gastrointestinal symptoms diminish further, but nutritional problems emerge more strongly. Gallbladder attacks are common unless the patient is on prophylactic medicine to prevent gallstone formation. Worrisome symptoms such as persistent vomiting, which may require some sort of intervention, may be related to intestinal obstruction or rupture of staples. Significant hypoglycemia (low blood glucose values) may develop in more than 5 percent of people, though this can usually be managed with nutrition counseling.

After the one-year mark, the major nutritional problems include anemia and osteoporosis. Over the years, a small percentage of people have developed neurological symptoms that probably are related to subtle nutritional deficiencies of multiple vitamins and minerals. Most commonly these symptoms are numbness and tingling of the feet due to neuropathy, ataxia or unsteadiness, and loss of cognitive function. Psychiatric symptoms that probably are multifactorial include depression, eating disorders, and suicide. Over ten years, various types of complications related to the surgery are seen in more than 50 percent of patients.

*Michelle was a thirty-seven-year-old nurse who had struggled with her weight since high school. She had successfully lost substantial amounts of weight on several occasions, but had enormous difficulty maintaining her weight losses. On her last effort, she had lost 60 pounds while participating in the Simple Diet program but had regained most of it while attending maintenance classes over the next year.*

*After appropriate guidance and counseling, Michelle decided to have gastric bypass surgery. Before surgery she weighed 252 pounds at five feet five inches tall. Her surgery went well, and she lost weight nicely. She had difficulty taking vitamin pills but did not seek advice (we would have recommended liquid vitamin and mineral supplements). She also had some difficulty with gas after consuming dairy products, so she limited milk and yogurt in her diet.*

*After several years, Michelle was able to achieve and maintain a health-promoting weight of around 160 pounds. About nine years after surgery she developed back pain, especially when assisting patients with shifting around in bed in the intensive care unit. Medical evaluation indicated that she had severe osteoporosis and several lumbar vertebrae that had partially collapsed. With intensive treatment for osteoporosis as well as supplementation with calcium and vitamin D, her condition stabilized. Unfortunately, she had to transfer out of intensive care—with sixteen years of experience there—into another area that did not require heavy lifting.*

## Complications after Laparoscopic Adjustable Gastric Banding (LAGB)

LAGB surgery has much lower mortality than gastric bypass surgery, but tends to have more complications, especially ones that require further invasive procedures. During the short hospital stay, bleeding or infections may be seen, and complication rates in the hospital are about 11.5 percent, or one in nine.

During the first month, gastrointestinal problems such as nausea, vomiting, diarrhea, and regurgitation are commonly seen. The more troublesome symptoms that can occur include esophagitis (inflammation or irritation of the esophagus) in 29 percent of patients; dilation of the esophagus, 10 percent; dilation of the small stomach pouch, 15 percent; slippage or migration of the band, 5 percent; problems with the port (opening on the abdominal wall connecting tubing to lap-band), 7 percent; leakage of the band, 6 percent; and erosion of the band into the stomach, 1 percent. About 12 percent of individuals require another operation to correct one or more of these problems.

After the first year, problems are less frequent because the LAGB procedure does not decrease absorption of important vitamins and minerals; the main problems relate to the band wearing out. One of the problems with placing artificial materials into the intestinal cavity is that they wear out and need to be replaced. Replacement rates for gastric bands are about 15 percent in three years and 32 percent in seven years.[50, 51]

*Katherine was a forty-three-year-old hospital administrator who came back to see me after a second operation to revise her gastric bypass surgery. She had been referred to me for assessment before surgery by her bariatric surgeon. I had advised her that an intensive weight-loss program such as the Simple Diet was my treatment recommendation before having bariatric surgery. However, since she qualified for surgery at five feet four inches tall and 252 pounds, she elected to have bariatric surgery.*

*Katherine was one of the unlucky 3 to 5 percent of patients who required a second operation to correct or reverse a prior Roux-en-Y gastric bypass. After the gastric bypass, she had a severe problem with vomiting and was not able to maintain adequate intakes to sustain her nutritional status. Blood levels of protein, vitamins, and minerals dropped to dangerously low levels within a few months after surgery. The surgical team recommended that she have a surgical revision of her stomach and small intestine to restore normal function as far as possible.*

*After surgery she was able to resume eating and began gaining weight. When she returned to over 250 pounds, she came back to see me. A nutritional assessment indicated that her blood levels had returned to normal, and I felt comfortable in prescribing an energy-restricted diet. I coached her on the Simple Diet, and she began losing about 1 pound per week, our goal. For the first time, she began trying to walk twelve miles per week and found that she could actually consume a wide variety of fruits and vegetables. At office visits she would regale me with recipes for acorn squash casseroles and blackberry puddings. Over six months of follow-up, she lost 30 pounds and was committed to this program the last time I saw her.*

# Comparative Weight Losses

The Swedish Obesity Study is one of the best studies of the long-term effects of bariatric surgery. The figure below compares weight loss after bariatric surgery reported from Sweden with our observations from the 100-Pound Club, many of whom followed a Simple Diet approach.[52] These 118 severely obese individuals lost an average of 135 pounds over a period of about one year. At six years they were keeping off 66 pounds. With gastric bypass surgery, individuals lost 85 pounds and were keeping off 69 pounds at six years. The difference between a diet and surgery after six years was less than three pounds. With LAGB, initial weight loss was 67 pounds and maintenance of weight loss at 6 years was 45 pounds. Compare the weight loss and then the risks, and tell me which one you would choose.

Bariatric surgery provides an opportunity for severely obese individuals to lose substantial amounts of weight and, on average, they remain slightly obese after completing their weight loss. The risk of death is in the same range as for similar surgical

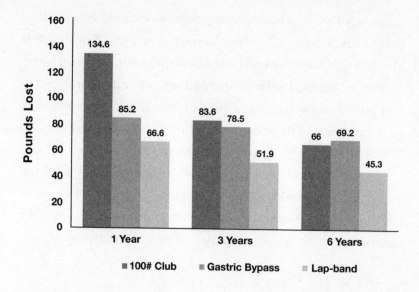

procedures of this magnitude involving patients with severe obesity. The risks for major complications are very high, and almost everyone has substantial gastrointestinal symptoms for as long as the surgically induced gastrointestinal alterations are maintained.

If you are more than 80 pounds overweight (have a BMI greater than 35 kg/m$^2$), you may qualify for bariatric surgery. However, you should consider the following: The risk of death is about one in sixty-three (1.6 percent). If you have family members who depend on you, this may be an unacceptable risk. The risks of substantial side effects during the first year are very high, and reoperations and additional hospitalizations also may be burdensome. It is likely that you will have gastrointestinal side effects indefinitely and will not be able to enjoy eating on special occasions.

The Simple Diet offers a much safer and probably more effective strategy for empowering you to achieve and maintain a health-protective weight. While it requires a substantial commitment of effort and time, your out-of-pocket expenses will be substantially lower than for bariatric surgery. The lifestyle changes will have far-reaching effects on your health. The increases in physical activity, increased fruit and vegetable consumption, and selection of foods lower in fat and sugar will have further health benefits in terms of reducing risk for cardiovascular disease, diabetes, and cancer.

My recommendation is that before opting for any of the available weight-loss surgeries, you make a serious twelve-week commitment to the Simple Diet to determine how effective this approach can be for your health and weight management.

# Beyond Weight Loss: Simple Lifetime Health

Y ou now have read all about the Simple Diet and are
ready to embark on a journey that will change your life.
Many of you may have already started and lost significant amounts of weight. Some of you have already reached your
goals. I have formulated the Simple Diet to help you keep the
number on the scale where you want it to be. But beyond weight
loss, I want to help you attain and maintain good health.

The steps you have taken on the Simple Diet have helped you
to lose weight and keep it off. Now I want to send you toward a
future of good health.

## You Are in Charge of Your Health

You are in charge of your health. All of us have genes that increase our risks for some health problems, such as heart dis-

ease, diabetes, or cancer. We can't change our genetic makeup, but we *can* reduce risks for almost all diseases through healthy lifestyle practices. Let's say that there is a strong history of diabetes in your family. You can reduce your risk of developing diabetes to almost *zero* by maintaining a lean body weight, being physically active, and eating well. You can reduce your risk of heart attack by 82 percent by not smoking, being trim and fit, and eating healthfully.[53]

You hold in your hands the ability to reduce your risk for heart disease, diabetes, high blood pressure, cancer, Alzheimer's disease, and many other diseases. I'll outline for you some of the elements that you have control over that will allow you to dramatically reduce or eliminate risks for most Western diseases.

## Dimensions of Health

Health management has four dimensions: physical, mental, emotional, and spiritual. These four are like the legs of a chair that support your health. The physical dimension includes being physically fit, achieving a health-promoting weight, and following the Simple Lifetime Diet. The mental dimension means having an active mind. As with your muscles, if you don't use your brain cells, their function declines. Emotional health involves appropriate management of stress, anxiety, and mood. Getting a full night's rest contributes to mental, physical, and emotional health. The spiritual dimension of health management requires having a sense of purpose, priorities, and motivation.

# The Physical Dimension: A Healthy Lifestyle Reduces Disease Risk

Extensive research documents that health-promoting lifestyle patterns may decrease the risk of heart disease by 82 percent, diabetes by 90 percent, hypertension by 60 percent, and cancer by 50 percent.[54] These lifestyle practices include eating an optimal diet, developing a fitness regimen to keep you trim and fit, and having good stress management practices. Overweight individuals have higher risks for heart disease, high blood pressure, diabetes, and certain cancers, especially breast and colon cancers. Excessive body fat creates a chronic inflammatory state and increased susceptibility to infections and autoimmune conditions such as fibromyalgia, lupus, and rheumatoid arthritis. Depression, psychosocial pain, and poor self-esteem commonly accompany obesity; these are aggravated by the multiple forms of prejudice and discrimination that obese individuals face. Finally, the life span of overweight and obese individuals is shortened, probably related to all the cardiovascular risk factors and lower levels of physical fitness.

## ▶ Health Benefits of Weight Loss

The good news is that most of these health problems can be eliminated or greatly reduced through lifestyle changes and weight loss. The health benefits of weight loss are too numerous to tabulate in this brief chapter. Are you taking any medications that you would like to get rid of? We recently reported that individuals who lost 42 pounds on the Simple Diet had major improvements in blood pressure, blood lipids, and diabetes. For patients taking medications for obesity-related conditions, average drug costs decreased from $237 per month to $65 per month.[55]

## ▶ Health Benefits of Physical Activity

Regular physical activity and maintaining a high level of fitness prolongs life, decreases risks for many major diseases, and enhances enjoyment of life. From head to toe, physical activity makes you more fit and healthy. Exercise perks up your brain, strengthens your heart, protects your liver, and enhances circulation. Heart disease remains the major cause of death for women and men in the United States. Physical activity strengthens the heart muscles and expands the blood vessels to facilitate greater blood flow to the heart. Physical activity also lowers blood pressure and fixes the blood lipids by decreasing blood total cholesterol, LDL cholesterol (the bad guys), and triglycerides, while increasing HDL cholesterol (the good guys).

How does exercise improve and protect brain function? On campus I frequently see students walking and texting at the same time. Many of my older friends walk cautiously and are concerned about stumbling or falling, while thirtysomething individuals walk briskly with little mental effort. Brisk walking requires much more mental work for my seventy-five-year-old friends than for their twenty-one-year-old grandchildren. So seniors who walk two miles daily at a decent pace are giving their muscles and their brains a much greater workout than seniors who exercise by changing channels with their television remote. Regular physical activity also contributes to stress management, relieves anxiety, and prevents depression. Thus, regular physical activity strongly supports physical and mental health.

## The Mental Dimension: Health Benefits of Brain Exercise

There is a broad consensus that seniors who use their brains for reading, crossword puzzles, problem solving, and social activities maintain cognitive function better than do individuals who spend many hours watching television daily. At the University of Kentucky, my good friends Dr. Bill Markesbery and Dr. David Snowdon spearheaded the Nun Study, which examined the relationship between a variety of brain-building activities and the pathology of the brains at autopsy. The Catholic sisters had been keenly interested in these studies and were eager to volunteer. Some very active "brain exercisers" and social sisters had advanced loss of brain tissue but functioned very well with their limited brain capacity; other sisters who had been less active socially and mentally had loss of cognitive function during life despite good preservation of brain tissue. In other words, if you don't use it, you lose it!

## The Emotional Dimension: Maintain a Positive Attitude

Maintaining your emotional equilibrium plays a vital role in dealing with the stress of everyday life, social interactions, and waves of anxiety or depression that we all have periodically. Hard-driving individuals with type A personalities have a higher risk for heart disease, while people who meditate regularly twice daily have a lower risk. Poor stress management increases risk for high blood pressure, stroke, and diabetes. Overweight individuals have more emotional challenges than slender individuals for a variety of reasons, some as a result of being overweight and some of which contribute to gaining even more weight. Regular exercise and meditation enhance stress management and assist in dealing with depression or anxiety.

A positive, upbeat attitude contributes to a healthy emotional state. Just as your smile tends to evoke a smile from others, a frown or dour demeanor may stimulate a sober attitude in response. Healthy, affirmative self-talk that displaces negative self-talk helps you with health and weight management and also contributes to a positive attitude. Positive attitudes attract positive responses from others.

# The Spiritual Dimension: Tapping into Spiritual Resources

The spiritual dimension gives our lives context and arises from our connection with ourselves and others. For some, spirituality takes the form of specific religious practices, meditation, prayer, or belief in a higher being. For others, spiritual fulfillment comes from communing with nature, enjoying music, or some other manner. My spiritual depth was enhanced when I practiced Transcendental Meditation and connected to the universal consciousness. My research indicates that having an all-embracing, universal outlook and an unselfish sense of responsibility gives life more perspective. Most individuals would be strengthened by developing a more secure spiritual perspective and drawing on the spiritual wisdom of ancient and modern faiths. All of us have a spiritual dimension that we can choose to nourish or let atrophy.

Meditation and prayer have many health benefits. For the past six years, I have done research on meditation, published two papers, and presented at international meetings. Transcendental Meditation (TM) has been the most extensively studied form of meditation and involves fifteen to twenty minutes of quiet meditation twice daily. I regularly practiced TM for two years as I began my research in this area. Our study documents that the regular practice of TM lowers blood pressure. Other research shows that TM also lowers serum cholesterol and risk for heart attack, perhaps through the well-documented effects on stress management and decreasing anxiety.

I also began practicing Centering Prayer about four years ago. Similar to TM, Centering Prayer is a rigorous discipline that involves at least twenty minutes of quiet meditation twice daily. For both meditation periods, you sit in a comfortable chair with your feet on the floor and focus on a religious word or phrase. My personal experience with Centering Prayer and my research leads me to conclude that Centering Prayer has the potential to provide the same health benefits as those achieved through TM.

Extensive research indicates that a variety of different meditation practices improve brain function, decrease anxiety, contribute to stress management, and have other health-promoting benefits.

# Your Simple Lifetime Diet

For more than thirty-five years, we have done research with high-fiber diets that focus on whole grains, beans, fruits, vegetables, and limited intakes of saturated fat and cholesterol from fatty beef, pork, and dairy products. The forerunner of the Simple Lifetime Diet has been shown to be effective in lowering blood pressure, fixing abnormal blood lipid numbers, and reversing or preventing diabetes. Thousands of research papers support the value of this type of diet for health preservation and disease prevention. The Simple Lifetime Diet is a health-promoting diet for everyone. A plethora of research by my team and that of other experts shows this is the optimal diet for health maintenance. MyPlate, the newest dietary advice recommended for everyone by the U.S. Department of Agriculture (www.choosemyplate.gov), shows three-quarters of a healthy plate being filled with vegetables, fruits, and grains—something we have been advocating for years with the Simple Lifetime Diet.

The Simple Diet, which has enabled you to lose to a health-promoting weight, is the most effective and safest nutrition and lifestyle approach to losing substantial weight. The First Phase focuses on intensive weight loss. The Second Phase focuses on developing a rhythm of habits that enable ongoing weight loss and health and weight management. The Simple Lifetime Diet is your diet for life. If some weight mysteriously accumulates, you can resume Phase Two of the Simple Diet, incorporating meal replacements, as I and many of my patients have done over the years.

The Simple Lifetime Diet encourages use of high-fiber, low-calorie fruits, vegetables, whole grains, and high-quality protein sources such as low-fat milk and cottage cheese, chicken or turkey breast, fish, and very lean cuts of beef or pork. You will focus on selecting foods primarily from the green zone of the Green Light Calorie Guide with judicious choices from the yellow zone (see chapter 10). You can jump-start your day with oatmeal, blueberries, and skim milk. Lunch could include a large green salad and a turkey sandwich with lettuce and tomato on whole wheat bread. Fresh fruit can be enjoyed mid-morning, at lunch, or midafternoon. Dinner could begin (as I try to always do) with a large green salad with tomatoes, followed by broiled fish, stir-fried mixed vegetables, and a fresh fruit salad. In my extensive world travels, I find that I can secure these food choices almost anywhere I go. You also should include soy foods such as soy milk, soy yogurt, tofu, or edamame in your diet because of their health benefits. Three to four ounces of white meat from chicken or turkey (baked or roasted without skin), fish, or tofu and 16 ounces of skim milk or low-fat soy milk products provide your protein. Try to minimize fat from all sources by using fat-free salad dressings, fat-free butter substitutes, and nonstick sprays. What follows is a sample three-day menu, and a seven-day menu is provided in the appendix (12.1, Seven-Day Sample Menu from the Simple Lifetime Diet). Appendices 10.2 and 10.3 give suggested numbers of servings to aim for from each of the calorie color zones for different body weights. Don't expect to find a lot of red zone and flashing red alert foods on this list!

## THREE-DAY MENU PLAN FOR THE SIMPLE
## LIFETIME DIET—2000 CALORIES PER DAY

| MEAL | DAY 1 | DAY 2 | DAY 3 |
|---|---|---|---|
| **Breakfast** | 1 cup cooked oatmeal with 1 cup non-fat soy milk and 1 cup blackberries and blueberries | ½ cup All Bran with 1 cup non-fat milk and 1 cup strawberries | 1 slice whole grain bread ½ cup non-fat plain yogurt with ½ cup mango |
| **Snack** | 1 cup raw vegetables (red peppers, celery, cherry tomatoes, carrots) with 1 tbsp. fat-free ranch dressing | 1 peach | Banana shake mix with 1 cup non-fat soy milk, 1 banana, ice cubes, and sweetener |
| **Lunch** | 1 cup black bean chili 1 slice whole grain toast 1 pear 1 cup non-fat yogurt | 1 cup shrimp pasta salad (⅔ cup whole wheat pasta, 2 oz. shrimp, celery, green pepper, and fat-free dressing) 3 cups spinach and mixed green salad with 1 tbsp. fat-free dressing 1 cup grilled asparagus 1 cup non-fat milk | 1 cup white bean and barley soup 2 cups baked summer squash 1 cup watermelon 1 cup non-fat milk |
| **Snack** | 1 orange | ¼ cup dry roasted soy nuts | 1 cup raw baby carrots with ¼ cup cottage cheese |
| **Dinner** | 3 cups mixed green salad with fat-free dressing 4 oz. grilled salmon 1 cup new red potatoes, boiled 1 cup oriental stir-fry vegetables sliced strawberries with 4 oz. low-fat soy milk and sweetener | 2 cups steamed mixed vegetables (broccoli, cauliflower, and carrots) 3 oz. marinated flank steak kebobs with mushrooms and cherry tomatoes ⅓ cup brown rice 1 clementine | Chicken bean taco (3 oz. cooked skinless chicken breast, ⅓ cup beans, corn tortilla, onion, green pepper, tomatoes, and lettuce) 1 cup green beans 1 cup cantaloupe |
| **Snack** | ½ cup Raisin Bran with ½ cup non-fat soy milk | 1 cup sugar-free pudding made with non-fat milk, mixed with ½ cup Flax Plus multigrain cereal | 1 cup cooked oat bran cereal with ½ cup non-fat soy milk |

"I can use the Simple Lifetime
Diet and consume five servings
of fruits and vegetables, three
servings of whole grains, and
select low-fat protein choices."

## Your Simple Lifetime Fitness Plan

You do not have to be skinny to be fit. While you want to achieve a health-promoting weight, you can become more fit while making progress toward your goal weight. During the First Phase (intensive weight loss), while you are focusing on losing down to your health-promoting weight, you should begin developing and tailoring your fitness program that you will follow indefinitely.

Fitness involves the three elements described in chapter 6. First is cardiovascular fitness. This is achieved by increasing physical activity in any shape or form. Walking is the most widely recommended physical activity because most people can walk, it can be done anywhere, and it does not require special equipment. Furthermore, walking is associated with less down time from injuries than running, cycling, and other more vigorous activities. The more miles you log per week, the lower your risk for cardiovascular disease, diabetes, and breast cancer.

Cardiovascular fitness can include but does not require aerobic activities such as brisk walking, water aerobics, running, swimming, and using elliptical machines and recumbent bicycles. In these activities, you increase your heart rate to 65 to 85 percent of the maximum rate. The table on page 101 in chapter 6 gives the desirable heart rate ranges for different ages. Aerobic fitness appears to confer an additional health protective benefit above that achieved with leisurely walking.

Total amounts of walking and the vigorousness of the walk (slow versus fast pace) have an important effect on the risk for heart attack. Women who do minimal amounts of walking at a slow pace are shown to have no significant change in heart attack risk. Women who do moderate amounts of walking at a slow pace have a 22 percent reduction in heart attack rate. Those who do large amounts of walking at a slow pace have a 29 percent reduction in risk. Moderate amounts of walking at a moderate pace reduced risk by 28 percent.[56] But minimal amounts of walking at a vigorous, fast pace substantially reduced risk. The greatest risk reduction for heart attacks is seen in fast walkers who do the largest amount of walking (using the recommended race-walking style). So, as in other areas of health behaviors, the more, the better.

The second element of fitness, strength training, confers additional health benefits, but these are difficult to quantify. For many years, I walked more than fourteen miles per week but did not work on my upper body strength. I feel much better now that I am doing weight training three days per week. Most of us use our biceps but let our triceps get flabby. This results in the "wings" under the arms that we see, especially in middle-aged or older women. Flabby muscles do not take up glucose readily and contribute to the risk for diabetes that 50 percent of Americans are subject to.

Stretching, the third element of fitness, keeps your muscles and tendons in prime shape to minimize injury. At my late age, I began stretching regularly last year and find that my muscles and tendons complain less when I do my 4.5-mile walk or participate in forty-five minutes of vigorous weight training in the gym.

You will need to develop your own fitness program and tailor it to your needs, enjoyment, and capability. A trainer at the gym or a personal trainer can give you guidance on this. However, you will need to commit about sixty minutes per day (six days a week) to achieve these goals.

The table below is my Guide to Total Fitness. After extensive research and trying a number of regimens, I have outlined a balanced approach to cardiovascular fitness, weight training, and stretching. Walking probably should account for about 50 percent of your activity because it is easy to do and can be done in short stretches during the day or with enjoyable longer walks.

## DR. ANDERSON'S GUIDE TO TOTAL FITNESS

| CATEGORY | ACTIVITY | SCHEDULE | MINUTES PER WEEK (CALORIES BURNED PER WEEK*) |
|---|---|---|---|
| Cardiovascular Fitness | Walking<br>Exercise bike<br>Aerobic exercise | 2 miles, 4 days a week<br><br>20 minutes, 3 days a week | 140 minutes (1,087 calories)<br>60 minutes (800 calories) |
| Weight training | Weight machines or hand weights | Use 18 machines, 15 repetitions, 3 days a week | 120 minutes (800 calories |
| Stretching | Stretching at home | 8 stretches, 15 seconds each, 6 days a week | 30 minutes (150 calories) |
| Total | | | 350 minutes (2,837 calories) |

* Calories estimated for a 200-pound individual. Calorie values for the four activities for a 150-pound person are (top to bottom) 815, 600, 600, 113, and 2,125 for total.

For optimal cardiovascular fitness, you should spend about 20 percent of your effort on aerobic exercise where your heart rate reaches a minimum of 65 percent of your maximum target rate. It is desirable to do weight training three days per week but no more. This can be done with weight machines at a gym or with hand weights at home. Weight training should represent about 25 percent of your fitness effort. Finally, you should do muscle stretching almost daily. These should be done after, and not before, your more vigorous exercises. Reaching these targets will represent burning about 2,800 calories for a 200-pound individual. After your weight loss from 200 pounds to a trim 150 pounds, you will burn about 25 percent fewer calories for these activities, but still will exceed our target of burning more than 2,000 calories per week in physical activity. I hope you are excited about getting started on these important health-promoting activities.

"Because of their health benefits, I will exercise regularly with cardiovascular activities, weight training, and stretching."

## Your Simple Lifetime Positive Outlook

An optimistic attitude and positive self-talk will be extremely helpful as you continue the Simple Lifetime Diet. These positive behaviors integrate the emotional, mental, and spiritual dimensions. Two of the best ways to make these behaviors work for you are through proactively developing a positive self-talk vocabulary and through meditation.

Positive thinking and self-talk can be developed to displace much of the negative self-talk chatter that our brains maintain continuously. Each time you catch yourself saying something negative, reframe it and replace it with a positive statement. Family members, friends, and others sometimes make negative statements that our brains like to keep repeating. For example, my colleagues tell me, "Jim, your office is a mess. I don't see how you can work with papers scattered all over the room." My taskmaster left brain tries to keep repeating this. But I do not accept it. I tell myself, "I am a very productive person and I focus on the task that has the highest priority." As another example, I love Krispy Kreme doughnuts. When I enter a store that has a doughnut showcase, I say, "I can walk past a Krispy Kreme showcase without hesitating," and I do.

To displace negative self-talk, you need to develop positive statements, write them down, say them aloud, and then repeat them again silently so they become your predominant thoughts. You will find more guidance in the appendix (3.2, Jump-Start Your Self-Talk).

"I can maintain an optimistic attitude and practice positive, affirming self-talk."

# Taking Charge of Your Health

You hold your health in your own hands now, as you choose to dedicate time and effort to intensive weight loss, and later, as you adopt healthy lifetime habits that provide solutions to Western diseases. By following the advice in this book, you can prevent, control, or even reverse many diseases and medical conditions. What's more, you will look and feel better, enjoy life more, and set a positive example for those around you.

You are not stuck with weight decisions made by your genes; you have choices. Choosing the Simple Diet and the Simple Lifetime Diet will help you live longer—and live better.

"I am committed to the Simple Lifetime Diet nutrition, physical activity, and positive outlook plans."

Appendices

# BODY MASS INDEX VALUES

To use the table, find the appropriate height in the left-hand column labeled Height. Move across to a given weight (in pounds). The number at the top of the column is the BMI at that height and weight. Pounds have been rounded off.

| BMI | 19 | 20 | 21 | 22 | 23 | 24 | 25 | 26 | 27 | 28 | 29 | 30 | 31 | 32 | 33 | 34 | 35 |
|---|---|---|---|---|---|---|---|---|---|---|---|---|---|---|---|---|---|
| HEIGHT (INCHES) | BODY WEIGHT (POUNDS) | | | | | | | | | | | | | | | | |
| 58 | 91 | 96 | 100 | 105 | 110 | 115 | 119 | 124 | 129 | 134 | 138 | 143 | 148 | 153 | 158 | 162 | 167 |
| 59 | 94 | 99 | 104 | 109 | 114 | 119 | 124 | 128 | 133 | 138 | 143 | 148 | 153 | 158 | 163 | 168 | 173 |
| 60 | 97 | 102 | 107 | 112 | 118 | 123 | 128 | 133 | 138 | 143 | 148 | 153 | 158 | 163 | 168 | 174 | 179 |
| 61 | 100 | 106 | 111 | 116 | 122 | 127 | 132 | 137 | 143 | 148 | 153 | 158 | 164 | 169 | 174 | 180 | 185 |
| 62 | 104 | 109 | 115 | 120 | 126 | 131 | 136 | 142 | 147 | 153 | 158 | 164 | 169 | 175 | 180 | 186 | 191 |
| 63 | 107 | 113 | 118 | 124 | 130 | 135 | 141 | 146 | 152 | 158 | 163 | 169 | 175 | 180 | 186 | 191 | 197 |
| 64 | 110 | 116 | 122 | 128 | 134 | 140 | 145 | 151 | 157 | 163 | 169 | 174 | 180 | 186 | 192 | 197 | 204 |
| 65 | 114 | 120 | 126 | 132 | 138 | 144 | 150 | 156 | 162 | 168 | 174 | 180 | 186 | 192 | 198 | 204 | 210 |
| 66 | 118 | 124 | 130 | 136 | 142 | 148 | 155 | 161 | 167 | 173 | 179 | 186 | 192 | 198 | 204 | 210 | 216 |
| 67 | 121 | 127 | 134 | 140 | 146 | 153 | 159 | 166 | 172 | 178 | 185 | 191 | 198 | 204 | 211 | 217 | 223 |
| 68 | 125 | 131 | 138 | 144 | 151 | 158 | 164 | 171 | 177 | 184 | 190 | 197 | 203 | 210 | 216 | 223 | 230 |
| 69 | 128 | 135 | 142 | 149 | 155 | 162 | 169 | 176 | 182 | 189 | 196 | 203 | 209 | 216 | 223 | 230 | 236 |
| 70 | 132 | 139 | 146 | 153 | 160 | 167 | 174 | 181 | 188 | 195 | 202 | 209 | 216 | 222 | 229 | 236 | 243 |
| 71 | 136 | 143 | 150 | 157 | 165 | 172 | 179 | 186 | 193 | 200 | 208 | 215 | 222 | 229 | 236 | 243 | 250 |
| 72 | 140 | 147 | 154 | 162 | 169 | 177 | 184 | 191 | 199 | 206 | 213 | 221 | 228 | 235 | 242 | 250 | 258 |
| 73 | 144 | 151 | 159 | 166 | 174 | 182 | 189 | 197 | 204 | 212 | 219 | 227 | 235 | 242 | 250 | 257 | 265 |
| 74 | 148 | 155 | 163 | 171 | 179 | 186 | 194 | 202 | 210 | 218 | 225 | 233 | 241 | 249 | 256 | 264 | 272 |
| 75 | 152 | 160 | 168 | 176 | 184 | 192 | 200 | 208 | 216 | 224 | 232 | 240 | 248 | 256 | 264 | 272 | 279 |
| 76 | 156 | 164 | 172 | 180 | 189 | 197 | 205 | 213 | 221 | 230 | 238 | 246 | 254 | 263 | 271 | 279 | 287 |

BODY WEIGHT (POUNDS)

| BMI | 36 | 37 | 38 | 39 | 40 | 41 | 42 | 43 | 44 | 45 | 46 | 47 | 48 | 49 | 50 | 51 | 52 | 53 | 54 |
|---|---|---|---|---|---|---|---|---|---|---|---|---|---|---|---|---|---|---|---|
| **HEIGHT (INCHES)** | | | | | | | | | | | | | | | | | | | |
| 58 | 172 | 177 | 181 | 186 | 191 | 196 | 201 | 205 | 210 | 215 | 220 | 224 | 229 | 234 | 239 | 244 | 248 | 253 | 258 |
| 59 | 178 | 183 | 188 | 193 | 198 | 203 | 208 | 212 | 217 | 222 | 227 | 232 | 237 | 242 | 247 | 252 | 257 | 262 | 267 |
| 60 | 184 | 189 | 194 | 199 | 204 | 209 | 215 | 220 | 225 | 230 | 235 | 240 | 245 | 250 | 255 | 261 | 266 | 271 | 276 |
| 61 | 190 | 195 | 201 | 206 | 211 | 217 | 222 | 227 | 232 | 238 | 243 | 248 | 254 | 259 | 264 | 269 | 275 | 280 | 285 |
| 62 | 196 | 202 | 207 | 213 | 218 | 224 | 229 | 235 | 240 | 246 | 251 | 256 | 262 | 267 | 273 | 278 | 284 | 289 | 295 |
| 63 | 203 | 208 | 214 | 220 | 225 | 231 | 237 | 242 | 248 | 254 | 259 | 265 | 270 | 278 | 282 | 287 | 293 | 299 | 304 |
| 64 | 209 | 215 | 221 | 227 | 232 | 238 | 244 | 250 | 256 | 262 | 267 | 273 | 279 | 285 | 291 | 296 | 302 | 308 | 314 |
| 65 | 216 | 222 | 228 | 234 | 240 | 246 | 252 | 258 | 264 | 270 | 276 | 282 | 288 | 294 | 300 | 306 | 312 | 318 | 324 |
| 66 | 223 | 229 | 236 | 241 | 247 | 253 | 260 | 266 | 272 | 278 | 284 | 291 | 297 | 303 | 309 | 315 | 322 | 328 | 334 |
| 67 | 230 | 236 | 243 | 249 | 255 | 261 | 268 | 274 | 280 | 287 | 293 | 299 | 306 | 312 | 319 | 325 | 331 | 338 | 344 |
| 68 | 236 | 243 | 249 | 256 | 262 | 269 | 276 | 282 | 289 | 295 | 302 | 308 | 315 | 322 | 328 | 335 | 341 | 348 | 354 |
| 69 | 243 | 250 | 257 | 263 | 270 | 277 | 284 | 291 | 297 | 304 | 311 | 318 | 324 | 331 | 338 | 345 | 351 | 358 | 365 |
| 70 | 250 | 257 | 264 | 271 | 278 | 285 | 292 | 299 | 306 | 313 | 320 | 327 | 334 | 341 | 348 | 355 | 362 | 369 | 376 |
| 71 | 257 | 265 | 272 | 279 | 286 | 293 | 301 | 308 | 315 | 322 | 329 | 338 | 343 | 351 | 358 | 365 | 372 | 379 | 386 |
| 72 | 265 | 272 | 279 | 287 | 294 | 302 | 309 | 316 | 324 | 331 | 338 | 346 | 353 | 361 | 368 | 375 | 383 | 390 | 397 |
| 73 | 272 | 280 | 288 | 295 | 302 | 310 | 318 | 325 | 333 | 340 | 348 | 355 | 363 | 371 | 378 | 386 | 393 | 401 | 408 |
| 74 | 280 | 287 | 295 | 303 | 311 | 319 | 326 | 334 | 342 | 350 | 358 | 365 | 373 | 381 | 389 | 396 | 404 | 412 | 420 |
| 75 | 287 | 295 | 303 | 311 | 319 | 327 | 335 | 343 | 351 | 359 | 367 | 375 | 383 | 391 | 399 | 407 | 415 | 423 | 431 |
| 76 | 295 | 304 | 312 | 320 | 328 | 336 | 344 | 353 | 361 | 369 | 377 | 385 | 394 | 402 | 410 | 418 | 426 | 435 | 443 |

Adapted from the National Heart, Lung, and Blood Institute, "Clinical Guidelines on Identification, Evaluation, and Treatment of Overweight and Obesity in Adults: The Evidence Report," NIH Publication No. 98-4083, September 1998.

Jump-Start Your Self-Talk

Positive, affirmative self-talk contributes importantly to health and weight management. The left brain is the dominant side for most people. The left brain is task-oriented and a relentless taskmaster. It reminds us of our shortcomings, often in negative ways such as "I am always late," "I am so disorganized," "I can't control my eating at a buffet," and "I can't resist Rocky Road ice cream." The right brain is the creative, imaginative, more relaxed side of the brain that acts like a loving, maternal figure that is positive and encouraging. It makes statements like "I am in charge of my schedule and can be on time or early for events, "I am a productive individual—I prioritize my work and focus on the most important task," "I can make healthy choices and eat moderately at a buffet," and "I can have a child's cup of mango sorbet in an ice-cream shop." The left brain takes charge of our thinking during waking hours and often does not let a word from the right brain be voiced. However, you can develop your right brain's statements and let them be heard.[57, 58]

This process will help you develop positive, affirming self-talk to replace negative statements. First, identify the positive statements that will help you in specific areas; examples are given below. Second, write the statements down. Third, read the statements aloud, and then again silently. Say them to yourself frequently. Fourth, when negative statements come up, like "I can't control my eating," replace them with positive ones, like "I can make healthy choices and eat moderately." Here are some positive self-talk statements in specific areas. Personalize them, write them down (include a current one on each Daily Progress and Weekly Summary Chart), and practice, practice, practice.

## ▶ General Goals

I am committed to improving my health and enjoyment of life through meeting goals related to diet, exercise, and record-keeping.

I set goals and I reach them. I know what my priorities are and they guide all my activities.

Each day I awake with a thankful, positive attitude. I make plans and I follow them.

I respect who I am and I maintain a healthy, can-do attitude.

## ▶ Simple Diet Goals

I can lose to my goal weight using three shakes and two entrées daily.

I am investing in my health and weight by eating at least five servings of fruits and vegetables daily.

I can decrease my need to snack and improve my rate of weight loss by consuming a large volume of fluids daily.

I appreciate _____'s willingness to support me on the Simple Diet; I will share my progress weekly.

## ▶ Fitness Goals

I can increase my daily physical activity and improve my health by _____(walking, swimming, going to the gym, or whatever you plan to do).

I exercise regularly and I enjoy it; this is a natural part of my day.

I schedule my day so that exercise is an integral part of what I do.

When I exercise, I am pleased with myself. I am doing a great job maintaining these healthy behaviors.

# DAILY PROGRESS CHART

DATE:

START OF WEEK WEIGHT:

| DAY | SHAKES | ENTRÉES | FRUITS/ VEGETABLES | BARS | ON THE DIET* | CONSUMED SEFV** | PHYSICAL ACTIVITY |
|---|---|---|---|---|---|---|---|
| M | | | | | | | |
| Tu | | | | | | | |
| W | | | | | | | |
| Th | | | | | | | |
| F | | | | | | | |
| Sa | | | | | | | |
| Su | | | | | | | |
| Total | | | | | | | |

*Consumed only meal replacements, bars, fruits, and vegetables and no other caloric items

** Consumed at least three shakes, two entrées, and five fruits and vegetables (SEFV)

**Self-talk:** I can _____

# WEEKLY SUMMARY CHART

**BEGINNING DATE:**
**BEGINNING WEIGHT:**

| WEEK | SHAKES | ENTRÉES | FRUITS/ VEGETABLES | BARS | ON THE DIET* | CONSUMED SEFV** | PHYSICAL ACTIVITY | WEIGHT |
|------|--------|---------|--------------------|------|--------------|-----------------|-------------------|--------|
| 1 | | | | | | | | |
| 2 | | | | | | | | |
| 3 | | | | | | | | |
| 4 | | | | | | | | |
| 5 | | | | | | | | |
| 6 | | | | | | | | |
| 7 | | | | | | | | |
| 8 | | | | | | | | |
| 9 | | | | | | | | |
| 10 | | | | | | | | |
| 11 | | | | | | | | |
| 12 | | | | | | | | |
| 13 | | | | | | | | |
| 14 | | | | | | | | |
| 15 | | | | | | | | |
| 16 | | | | | | | | |

*Consumed only meal replacements, bars, fruits, and vegetables and no other caloric items
** Consumed at least three shakes, two entrées, and five fruits and vegetables (SEFV)

**Self-talk:** I can _____

Recommended Shakes

These are just some of the many shakes meeting nutrition guidelines: 100 to 200 calories, 10 to 26 grams of protein, and less than 6 grams of fat.

**Equate**
- Creamy Milk Chocolate*
- French Vanilla*
- Strawberries 'n Cream*

**GNC**
- Rich Chocolate #
- Swiss Chocolate *#
- French Vanilla #
- Vanilla Bean *#
- Cookies & Cream #
- Strawberries & Cream *#
- Blueberries & Cream #

**Naturade Total Soy**
- Chocolate #
- Vanilla #
- French Vanilla #
- Bavarian Chocolate #
- Strawberry Creme #

**Revival Soy (unsweetened or with sucralose sweetener)**
- Chocolate Daydream #
- Vanilla Pleasure #
- Strawberry Smile #
- Banana Blessings #
- Strawberry Banana Bliss #

- Blueberry Blush #
- Just Peachy! #
- Cappuccino Comfort #
- Plain Soy #

**Slim-Fast**
- Creamy Milk Chocolate *#
- Rich Chocolate Royale *#
- High Protein Extra Creamy Chocolate *#
- French Vanilla *#
- High Protein Creamy Vanilla #
- Strawberries N' Cream*
- Strawberry Supreme #
- Cappuccino Delight*

**Slim-Rite (Kroger brand)**
- Creamy Milk Chocolate*
- Chocolate*
- French Vanilla*
- Original Chocolate Royale*
- Strawberry Cream*
- Vanilla*

**Special K Protein Shakes**
- Milk Chocolate*
- French Vanilla*
- Strawberry*

* come premixed in liquid form in cans or bottles
# come in powder form and need to be mixed with milk or other fluid

Recommended Entrées

These are just some of the many entrées meeting nutrition guidelines: 140 to 300 calories, 10 to 25 grams of protein, and less than 9 grams of fat.

## Banquet
- Cheese Smothered Charbroiled Patties
- Chicken Nuggets and Fries
- Chicken Pasta Marinara
- Chicken with Dumplings
- Creamy Broccoli, Chicken & Cheese with Rice
- Salisbury Steak Meal

## Healthy Choice

### All Natural Entrées
- Lobster Cheese Ravioli
- Portabella Marsala Pasta
- Portabella Spinach Parmesan
- Tortellini Primavera Parmesan

### Café Steamers
- Balsamic Garlic Chicken
- Beef Teriyaki
- Cajun Style Chicken & Shrimp
- Chicken Red Pepper Alfredo
- Grilled Basil Chicken
- Grilled Chicken Marinara
- Grilled Whiskey Steak
- Kung Pao Chicken
- Lemon Garlic Chicken and Shrimp
- Lemongrass Chicken & Shrimp
- Roasted Beef Merlot
- Roasted Chicken Fresca
- Roasted Chicken Marsala
- Sweet & Spicy Orange Zest Chicken
- Thai-Style Chicken & Vegetables

### Complete Meals
- Beef Bourbon Dijon
- Beef Pot Roast
- Beef Tips Portobello
- Chicken Pesto Alfredo
- Country Herb Chicken
- Golden Roasted Turkey Breast
- Lemon Pepper Fish
- Oven Roasted Chicken
- Spicy Shrimp Diavolo
- Turkey Marsala

### Fresh Mixers
- Balsamic Vegetable Medley
- Creamy Tomato Basil Penne
- Penne & Roasted Red Pepper Alfredo
- Rotini & Zesty Marinara Sauce

- Steak Portobello

*Select Entrées*
- Bacon & Smokey Cheddar Chicken
- Chicken Alfredo Florentine
- Pineapple Chicken
- Ravioli Florentine Marinara
- Salisbury Steak
- Slow-Roasted Turkey Medallions

*Steaming Entrées*
- Chicken Romano Fresca
- Garlic Herb Shrimp
- Honey Balsamic Chicken
- Lemon Herb Chicken
- Roasted Chicken Verde
- Rosemary Chicken & Sweet Potatoes
- Sesame Glazed Chicken

**Kashi Frozen Entrées**
- Chicken Florentine
- Chicken Pasta Pomodoro
- Lemongrass Coconut Chicken
- Red Curry Chicken

**Lean Cuisine**

*Cafe Cuisine*
- Beef and Broccoli
- Beef Portabello
- Chicken with Almonds
- Chicken and Vegetables
- Chicken Carbonara
- Chicken Marsala
- Chicken with Basil Cream Sauce
- Fiesta Grilled Chicken

- Glazed Chicken
- Grilled Chicken Caesar
- Lemon Pepper Fish
- Orange Chicken
- Parmesan Crusted Fish
- Roasted Garlic Chicken
- Shrimp Alfredo
- Shrimp and Angel Hair Pasta
- Steak Tips Portabello
- Sun-dried Tomato Pesto Chicken
- Sweet and Sour Chicken
- Thai-Style Chicken
- Three Cheese Stuffed Rigatoni
- Tortilla Crusted Fish

*Casual Cuisine*
- Fajita-style Chicken Spring Rolls
- Garlic Chicken Spring Rolls
- Mushroom Pizza
- Thai-Style Chicken Spring Rolls

*Comfort Cuisine*
- Baked Chicken
- Beef Pot Roast
- Chicken Parmesan
- Chicken with Lasagna Rollatini
- Glazed Turkey Tenderloins
- Herb Roasted Chicken
- Meatloaf with Mashed Potatoes
- Roasted Turkey and Vegetables
- Roasted Turkey Breast
- Salisbury Steak with Macaroni and Cheese

*Dinnertime Cuisine*
- Chicken Portabello
- Chicken Tuscan
- Lemon Garlic Shrimp
- Roasted Turkey Breast
- Salisbury Steak
- Steak Tips Dijon

*Market Creations*
- Asiago Cheese Tortelloni
- Chicken Alfredo
- Chicken Margherita
- Chicken Poblano
- Chicken Pot Stickers
- Garlic Chicken
- Mushroom Tortelloni
- Shanghai-Style Shrimp
- Shrimp Scampi
- Sweet & Spicy Ginger Chicken

*Simple Favorites*
- Alfredo Pasta with Chicken & Broccoli
- Baja-Style Chicken Quesadilla
- BBQ Chicken Ranch Quesadilla
- Cheddar Potatoes with Broccoli
- Cheese Ravioli
- Chicken Florentine Lasagna
- Chicken Chow Mein
- Chicken Enchilada Suiza
- Chicken Fettuccini
- Chicken Fried Rice
- Chicken Teriyaki Stir Fry
- Classic Macaroni and Beef
- Deluxe Cheddar Potato
- Four Cheese Cannelloni
- Linguine Carbonara
- Macaroni and Cheese
- Pasta Romano with Bacon

- Roasted Chicken with Lemon Pepper Fettuccini
- Santa Fe–Style Rice & Beans
- Spaghetti with Meat Sauce
- Spaghetti with Meatballs
- Stuffed Cabbage
- Swedish Meatballs with Pasta

*Spa Cuisine*
- Chicken in Peanut Sauce
- Chicken Mediterranean
- Ginger Garlic Stir Fry with Chicken
- Grilled Chicken Primavera
- Hunan Stir Fry with Beef
- Lemon Chicken
- Lemongrass Chicken
- Roasted Honey Chicken
- Rosemary Chicken
- Salmon with Basil
- Sesame Stir Fry with Chicken
- Szechuan-Style Stir Fry with Shrimp

## Michelina's

*Authentico*
- Four Cheese Lasagna
- Lasagna with Meat Sauce
- Pasta & Chicken
- Spaghetti with Meat Sauce

*Michelina's Lean Gourmet*
- Apple Cranberry Chicken
- Baked Ham & Cheese Snackers
- Baked Pepperoni Pizza Snackers
- Beef & Peppers
- Beef Supreme
- Chicken Alfredo Florentine

- Chicken & Pasta Bake
- Chicken Club Flatbread
- Creamy Rigatoni with Broccoli & Chicken
- Fettuccine Alfredo with Broccoli
- Five Cheese Lasagna
- Glazed Chicken
- Macaroni & Cheese with Jalapeno Peppers
- Mama's Pasta & Bacon Bake
- Meatloaf
- Penne Primavera
- Pepperoni Flatbread Pizza
- Salisbury Steak
- Santa Fe–Style Rice & Beans
- Sesame Chicken
- Shrimp Scampi
- Shrimp with Pasta & Vegetables
- Spinach & Ricotta Bake
- Three Cheese Chicken
- Three Cheese Ziti

*Zap'ems Gourmet*
- Angel Hair Pasta in Meat Sauce
- Fettuccine Alfredo
- Italian-style Vegetables & White Chicken
- Lasagna with Meat Sauce
- Macaroni & Beef
- Macaroni & Cheese with Cheddar and Romano
- Pasta & Chicken
- Rigatoni in Sauce with Broccoli & White Chicken

**Smart Ones Breakfast**
- Breakfast Quesadilla

- Canadian Style Bacon English Muffin Sandwich
- Cheesy Scramble with Hashbrowns
- Egg, Sausage and Cheese Smart Morning Wrap
- English Muffin Sandwich
- French Toast with Turkey Sausage
- Ham and Cheese Scramble
- Stuffed Breakfast Sandwich

**Smart Ones**
- Broccoli & Cheddar Roasted Potatoes
- Cheese Pizza Minis
- Chicken Quesadilla
- Chicken & Mushroom Florentine Smart Mini Wraps
- Chicken Carbonara
- Chicken Enchiladas Suiza
- Chicken Fettucini
- Chicken Marinara with Mozzarella Cheese Grilled Flatbread
- Chicken Marsala
- Chicken Oriental
- Chicken Parmesan
- Chicken Ranchero Smart Mini Wraps
- Chicken Santa Fe
- Cranberry Turkey Medallions
- Creamy Parmesan Chicken
- Creamy Rigatoni with Broccoli & Chicken
- Fettucini Alfredo
- Fiesta Quesadilla
- Home Style Beef Pot Roast
- Lasagna Bake with Meat Sauce

- Lemon Herb Chicken Piccata
- Macaroni & Cheese
- Meatloaf
- Mini Cheeseburgers
- Mini Rigatoni with Vodka Cream Sauce
- Pasta Primavera
- Pasta with Ricotta and Spinach
- Pepperoni Pizza Minis
- Ravioli Florentine
- Salisbury Steak (both 9 oz. and 9.5 oz.)
- Savory Steak & Ranch Grilled Flatbread
- Slow-Roasted Turkey Breast
- Spaghetti with Meat Sauce
- Spicy Szechuan Style Vegetable & Chicken
- Stuffed Turkey Breast
- Swedish Meatballs
- Sweet & Sour Chicken
- Teriyaki Chicken & Vegetables
- Thai Style Chicken & Rice Noodles
- Three Cheese Macaroni
- Three Cheese Ziti Marinara
- Traditional Lasagna with Meat Sauce
- Tuna Noodle Gratin
- Vegetable Pizza Minis

These are just some of the many bars meeting nutrition guidelines: 100 to 200 calories, 10 to 20 grams of protein, and less than 5 grams of fat.

**Balance Bars**
- Caramel Nut Blast
- Chocolate Peanut Butter
- Double Chocolate Brownie
- Mocha Chip
- S'mores
- Yogurt Honey Peanut

**GNC**

*FullBar Bars*
- Double Chocolate Cocoa Crisp

*ProCrunch Lite Bars*
- Chocolate Crisp

*Total Lean Bars*
- Peanut Butter Chocolate Chip
- Vanilla Zest

*WELLbeING be-NOURISHED Bars*
- Chocolate Soy Crisp
- Cinnamon Almond Crunch
- Strawberry Peanut Crunch

**Kashi GOLEAN Bars**
- Caramel Peanut
- Chocolate Almond
- Chocolate Caramel
- Chocolate Peanut
- Chocolate Pretzel
- Chocolate Turtle
- Cinnamon Coffee Cake
- Honey Almond Flax
- Honey Toasted 7 Grain
- Peanut Peanut Butter
- Pumpkin Spice Flax
- Roasted Almond Crunch
- Trail Mix

**Luna Bars**
- Berry Almond
- Blueberry Bliss
- Caramel Nut Brownie
- Chocolate Chunk
- Cookie Dough
- Chocolate Raspberry
- Chocolate Peppermint Stick
- Cookies 'n Cream Delight
- Iced Oatmeal Raisin
- LemonZest
- Nutz Over Chocolate
- Peanut Butter Cookie
- S'mores
- Toasted Nuts 'n Cranberry
- Vanilla Almond

### Optimum Energy Bars
- Blueberry Flax & Soy

### Pure Protein Bars
- Blueberry Crumb Cake
- Chewy Chocolate Chip
- Chocolate Deluxe
- Chocolate Peanut Butter
- Chocolate Peanut Caramel
- Peanut Marshmallow Eclipse
- Protein Revolution
- Strawberry Shortcake
- S'Mores

### Zone Perfect Nutrition Bars
- Blueberry
- Cashew Pretzel

- Chocolate Caramel Cluster
- Chocolate Chip Cookie Dough
- Dark Chocolate Almond
- Dark Chocolate Caramel Pecan
- Dark Chocolate Cookies N' Creme
- Dark Chocolate Strawberry
- Double Dark Chocolate
- Fudge Graham
- Peanut Butter Cookie Dough
- Strawberry Yogurt
- Trail Mix

# Appendix 4.4

Recommended Soups

Some soups meeting nutrition guidelines: 100 to 200 calories, 10 to 20 grams of protein, and less than 6 grams of fat.

## Healthy Choice (includes cans and microwavable bowls)

- Bean & Ham
- Chicken Tortilla
- Italian Wedding Style
- Split Pea & Ham
- Steak and Noodle
- Vegetable Beef

## LOW-, MODERATE-, AND HIGH-CALORIE
## CLASSIFICATION OF FRUITS

| LOW 40 CALORIES/SERVING (LESS THAN 13 CALORIES/OUNCE) | MODERATE 50 CALORIES/SERVING (13 TO 20 CALORIES/ OUNCE) | HIGH 50 CALORIES/SERVING (MORE THAN 20 CALORIES/OUNCE) |
|---|---|---|
| Serving size 1 cup | Serving size 1 cup | Serving size ½ cup |
| Cantaloupe | Apple | Avocado |
| Grapefruit | Apricot | Banana |
| Honeydew melon | Blackberries | Sweet cherries |
| Mandarin orange | Blueberries | |
| Papaya | Cranberries | |
| Peach | Grapes | |
| Strawberries | Kiwifruit | |
| Tangelo | Mango | |
| Tangerine | Nectarine | |
| Watermelon | Navel orange | |
| | Pear | |
| | Pineapple | |
| | Plum | |
| | Pomegranate | |
| | Raspberries | |

## LOW-, MODERATE-, AND HIGH-CALORIE
## CLASSIFICATION OF VEGETABLES

| LOW<br>25 CALORIES/SERVING (LESS THAN 10 CALORIES/OUNCE) | MODERATE<br>50 CALORIES/SERVING (10 TO 25 CALORIES/OUNCE) | HIGH<br>100 CALORIES/SERVING (MORE THAN 25 CALORIES/OUNCE) |
|---|---|---|
| Serving Size 1 cup | Serving Size ½ cup | Serving Size ½ cup |
| Asparagus | Alfalfa sprouts | Vegetarian beans |
| Beets | Yellow corn | White beans |
| Broccoli | Green lima beans | Black-eyed peas |
| Brussels sprouts | Peas | Garbanzo beans |
| Cabbage | | Kidney beans |
| Carrot | | Lentils |
| Cauliflower | | White potato |
| Celery | | Soybeans |
| Cucumber | | Sweet potato |
| Eggplant | | |
| Green beans | | |
| Kale | | |
| Kohlrabi | | |
| Lettuce | | |
| Mushrooms | | |
| Mustard greens | | |
| Okra | | |
| Onion | | |
| Bell pepper | | |
| Pumpkin | | |

| LOW 25 CALORIES/SERVING (LESS THAN 10 CALORIES/OUNCE) | MODERATE 50 CALORIES/SERVING (10 TO 25 CALORIES/OUNCE) | HIGH 100 CALORIES/SERVING (MORE THAN 25 CALORIES/OUNCE) |
|---|---|---|
| Red radish | | |
| Spinach | | |
| Acorn and zucchini squash | | |
| Summer and winter squash | | |
| Red tomato | | |
| Turnip greens | | |

## APPROXIMATE DAILY CALORIE, VOLUME, AND NUTRITION VALUES FOR THREE DIETS*

| DAILY NUTRITION INFORMATION | SIMPLE DIET | JENNY CRAIG | NUTRI-SYSTEM |
|---|---|---|---|
| Calories/day | 1153 | 1453 | 1525 |
| Carbohydrate, grams/day | 155 | 219 | 220 |
| Protein, grams/day | 95 | 81 | 78 |
| Fat, grams/day | 17 | 28 | 45 |
| Fiber, grams/day | 15 | 24 | 24 |
| Volume, calories/ounce | 13 | 22 | 23 |
| **GENERAL DIET INFORMATION** | | | |
| Desserts and snack foods available | bars | 23[a] | 34[b] |
| Non-portion-control foods[c] | Fruits; vegetables; condiments | Fruits; vegetables; juices; condiments; low-fat dairy; 11 sweets; nuts; olives | Fruits; vegetables; juices; condiments; 7 dairy; 31 proteins, breads; nuts |
| Minimum weekly product purchase requirement[d] | $49 | $127 | $60 |
| Food costs to follow minimum recommended intake weekly[e] | $12 | $21 | $32 |

*Calculated from seven-day menu plans developed from support guides for each of the diets.
[a] Includes bars, brownies, cake, candy, cheese puffs, chips, cookies, crisps, pretzels, snack mix.
[b] Includes bars, brownies, cake, cheesecake, cheese curls, chips, cookies, popcorn, pretzels, and twists.
[c] Because all three diets encourage controlling the serving sizes of foods (portion-control), the degree to which the diets permit inclusion of foods that are not pre-packaged in serving-sized portions is compared. All three diets encourage use of fruits, vegetables, and low-calorie condiments. Jenny Craig and Nutrisystem encourage use of a wide variety of foods (such as non-fat milk, juices, and nuts) that are not portion-controlled.
[d] Products: Minimum cost for purchase of shakes, entrées, and other food products recommended as minimum consumption weekly. Data based on food purchased in June 2010.
[e] Grocery costs to purchase minimum weekly needed fruits and vegetables (all diets); cheese and skim milk (Jenny Craig); and almonds, cottage cheese, oatmeal, skim milk, and whole wheat rolls (Nutrisystem).

## THE SIMPLE DIET SEVEN-DAY SAMPLE MENUS

| MEAL | SUNDAY | MONDAY | TUESDAY | WEDNESDAY | THURSDAY | FRIDAY | SATURDAY |
|---|---|---|---|---|---|---|---|
| **Breakfast** | Breakfast Quesadilla (Smart Ones), 1 grapefruit | Cappuccino Delight shake (Slim-Fast) | Rich Chocolate Royale shake (Slim-Fast) | Strawberries N' Cream shake (Slim-Fast), Honeydew melon | Creamy Milk Chocolate shake (Slim-Fast) | Strawberry shake (Special K) | Ham and Cheese Scramble (Smart Ones), 1 orange |
| **Snack** | Creamy Milk Chocolate shake (Slim-Fast) | Chocolate Daydream powder (Revival Soy) blended with 1 cup strawberries | Vanilla Bean powder (GNC) blended with 1 cup mixed berries | Vanilla Pleasure powder (Revival Soy) blended with 12 oz. diet soda | Rich Chocolate Royale powder (Slim-Fast) blended with ½ banana | Strawberry Smile powder (Revival Soy) blended with 1 cup frozen mixed fruit | French Vanilla powder (Slim-Fast) blended with 1 cup frozen strawberries |
| **Lunch** | Roasted Beef Merlot (Healthy Choice), ½ cup mashed potatoes, veggie dip*, 1 cup fruit salad | Chicken Quesadilla (Smart Ones), 1 cup carrots, 1 orange | Fettuccine Alfredo with Broccoli (Michelina's), 3 cups mixed salad with diet dressing, 1 peach | Cheese Ravioli (Lean Cuisine), veggie dip, 1 apple | Chicken Marsala (Smart Ones), 1 cup zucchini squash, 1 cup blueberries | Lemon Pepper Fish (Healthy Choice), 3 cups Mixed salad, 1 cup strawberries | Baked Chicken (Lean Cuisine), veggie dip, 1 cup watermelon |
| **Snack** | Blueberry Blush powder (Revival Soy) blended with 12 oz. diet soda | Creamy Milk Chocolate shake (Slim-Fast) | Strawberries 'n Cream shake (Equate) | Swiss Chocolate shake (GNC) | French Vanilla shake (Special K) | Creamy Milk Chocolate shake (Equate) | Just Peachy! powder (Revival Soy) blended with 12 oz. diet soda |

| MEAL | SUNDAY | MONDAY | TUESDAY | WEDNESDAY | THURSDAY | FRIDAY | SATURDAY |
|---|---|---|---|---|---|---|---|
| **Dinner** | Chicken Carbonara (Smart Ones), 1 cup asparagus, 1 nectarine | Roasted Garlic Chicken (Lean Cuisine), 3 cups mixed salad with diet dressing, 1 cup blueberries | Lasagna Bake with Meat Sauce (Smart Ones), Veggie dip, 1 cup cantaloupe | Chicken Mediterranean (Lean Cuisine), 1 cup broccoli, 1 cup raspberries | Salisbury Steak (Healthy Choice), 1 cup green beans, 1 papaya | Pepperoni Flatbread Pizza (Michelina's), Veggie dip, 1 cup grapes | Chicken Pesto Alfredo (Healthy Choice), 3 cups mixed salad with diet dressing, 1 cup blackberries |
| **Snack** | Swiss Chocolate powder (GNC) blended with 12 oz. diet soda | French Vanilla powder (Slim-Fast) blended with 12 oz. diet root beer | Banana Blessings powder (Revival Soy) blended with 12 oz. water | Vanilla Bean powder (GNC) blended with 12 oz. diet soda | Blueberry Blush powder (Revival Soy) blended with 12 oz. diet soda | French Vanilla shake (GNC) | Cookies & Cream powder (GNC) blended with 12 oz. diet 7-UP |

*Veggie dip: Select 2 cups of three to five vegetables (bell pepper, broccoli, baby carrots, cauliflower, celery, cherry tomatoes, cucumbers, or radishes); add 1 tbsp. fat-free dressing of your choice. Dip and enjoy.

A mazon (amazon.com) provides up-to-date guides for pedometers. The basic need is a pedometer that you can wear and that reliably measures your steps.

When you get your pedometer, calibrate it by walking one mile on the sidewalk, track, or gym and determine how many steps you take in a mile. Your pedometer should consistently measure the same number of steps every time you walk that mile or distance. Once you have determined how many steps per mile (about two thousand for the average person), estimate your miles walked daily by dividing your number of steps by two thousand or your own number of steps per mile.

I like simple pedometers that focus on measuring total steps. Fancier ones, often larger, will compute calories and have a memory of your number of steps each day for a week.

Currently I am using the highly rated Omron (HJ-112 Digital Pocket Pedometer), which has memory and also a security strap and can be carried in your pocket or bag. Omron has a variety of highly rated pedometers (http:www.pedometerusa.com/omron-pedometers). Accusplit also has an array of excellent pedometers (http://www.accusplit.com/).

# Appendix 6.2

## Recommended Exercise Guides

These are exercise and fitness books that I find helpful:

American College of Sports Medicine. *ASCN Fitness Book*. Third Edition (Champaign, IL: Human Kinetics, 2003).

Cooper, K. H. *The Aerobics Program for Total Well-Being* (New York: Bantam, 1982).

Hoeger, W. W. K., S. A. Hoeger. *Lifetime Physical Fitness and Wellness.* Ninth Edition. (Belmont, CA: Thomson Wadsworth, 2007).

Karpay, E. *The Everything Total Fitness Book* (Holbrook, MA: Adams Media Corp., 2000).

Peeke, P. *Body-for-LIFE for Women* (Emmaus, PA: Rodale Books, 2005).

Phillips, B., and M. D'Orso, *Body for Life* (New York: Harper Collins, 1999).

Meyers, C. *Walking: A Complete Guide to the Complete Exercise* (New York: Random House, 1992).

# FEATURES OF SOME WEIGHT-LOSS WEBSITES

| WEBSITE | SPARKPEOPLE.COM | STARTYOURDIET.COM | LIVESTRONG.COM | FATSECRET.COM | EVERYDAY HEALTH.COM | CALORIECOUNT.ABOUT.COM | EATTHIS.COM |
|---|---|---|---|---|---|---|---|
| Blog | x | x | x | | x | | |
| BMI Calculator/Tracker | x | x | x | | x | x | |
| Challenges | | x | x | x | | | |
| Daily Feedback and Charts | x | x | x | x | | x | |
| Daily Food Consumption | x | x | x | x | x | x | |
| Exercise Difficulty Level | | | x | x | x | x | |
| Exercise Tracker | x | x | x | x | x | x | |
| Fitness Demonstrations | x | | x | | | x | |
| Goals (set and track) | x | x | x | x | x | x | |
| Groups | x | | x | x | x | x | |
| Health Articles | x | x | x | | x | | x |

| WEBSITE | SPARKPEOPLE .COM | START YOURDIET.COM | LIVESTRONG .COM | FATSECRET .COM | EVERYDAY HEALTH.COM | CALORIECOUNT .ABOUT.COM | EATTHIS.COM |
|---|---|---|---|---|---|---|---|
| Inspirational/ Motivational Quotes | x | | | | | | |
| Journal | x | x | x | x | x | x | |
| Message Boards/ Forum | x | x | x | x | x | x | |
| Profile Page | x | x | x | x | x | x | |
| Post Pictures | x | x | x | x | x | x | |
| Success Stories | x | | | | | | |
| Tracks Body Measurements | x | x | | | | | |
| Trivia | x | | | | | x | x |
| Walking Route Map | x | | x | | | | |
| Water Consumption Tracker | x | x | x | | x | | |
| Weight-loss Graph | x | x | x | x | x | x | |
| Weight-loss Tips | x | x | | | x | | x |
| Membership Type | Free | $30/year | Free; upgrade $45/ year | Free | Free; premium $3/wk | Free | $20/year |

Summary of the Simple Diet for Your Doctor

# FIRST PHASE: INTENSIVE WEIGHT-LOSS PHASE (Until Healthy Weight Is Reached)
-- -- -- -- -- -- -- -- -- -- -- -- -- -- -- --

## ▶ The Six Keys of Intensive Weight Loss

1. Use at least five meal replacements daily (three shakes, two entrées).*

2. Eat at least five servings of fruits and vegetables daily (without added fat or sugar).

3. Add volume and variety (drink a minimum of eight 8-ounce glasses of noncaloric fluids daily; if needed, higher volume of shakes and lower-calorie choices).

4. Build up to burning 2,000 additional calories in physical activity weekly (about two to three miles, or thirty to forty-five minutes, of walking six days weekly).

5. Keep daily records of whether you've met or exceeded recommendations (for physical activity and servings of shakes, entrées, fruits, and vegetables).

6. Be accountable to someone (a family member, friend, or your doctor).

*Rationale for recommending meal replacements: reduce choices and replace other higher-calorie foods with low-calorie, nutritionally balanced foods in preportioned amounts. One-a-day multivitamin and mineral supplement use also recommended.

## ▶ Average Daily Composition of the Simple Diet

Calories: ≥ 1,200; Protein ≥ 80 grams

## ▶ Expected Rate of Weight Loss

Women (average 200 pounds): 11 pounds first four weeks, 1 to 3 pounds per week thereafter

Men (average 250 pounds): 16 pounds first four weeks, 1.5 to 3.5 pounds per week thereafter[59]

# SECOND PHASE: HEALTH AND WEIGHT MANAGEMENT PHASE (Minimum of Six Months)

Gradual introduction of a greater variety of healthy, low-fat foods

## ▶ The Six Keys of Health and Weight Management

1. Use at least two meal replacements (shakes or entrées) daily in combination with other low-fat foods.
2. Eat at least five servings of fruits and vegetables (without added fat or sugar) daily.
3. Add volume and variety (drink a minimum of eight 8-ounce glasses of noncaloric fluids daily

and choose lower-calorie foods, including very lean protein and whole grains).

4. Burn at least 2,000 additional calories in physical activity weekly (about two to three miles, or thirty to forty-five minutes of walking six days weekly).

5. Keep daily summaries of recommended food intake and physical activity.

6. Be accountable to someone (a family member, friend, or your doctor).

# FROM DR. ANDERSON TO YOUR DOCTOR:

James W. Anderson, MD, FACP, FACN, CNS, has done extensive research and clinical work using very-low-calorie diets (VLCDs) and low-calorie diets and published over one hundred scientific articles in this area. He established and directed the Health Management Resources (HMR) Program at the University of Kentucky, treating over five thousand patients over twenty-five years. This experience indicates that the Simple Diet is very safe and requires minimal medical supervision. Nevertheless, because obesity is associated with a number of risk factors that require periodic reassessment, he routinely encourages his patients to have the following evaluation before embarking on an intensive weight-loss program:

- Update history and medication list
- Update physical examination

- Obtain routine panel of twenty chemistry measurements, lipid profile, and complete blood count
- Assess and monitor these clinical conditions as indicated medically (I am available by e-mail to primary care providers at askdranderson@aol.com)
- Hypertension: As you know, blood pressure drops dramatically with weight loss. Because many patients substantially decrease their sodium intake when starting the diet, we routinely discontinue thiazide diuretics when they start the diet. Patients need to monitor their own blood pressure, be aware of the symptoms of orthostatic hypotension, and be coached in reduction of their other antihypertensive medications as they lose weight.
- Diabetes: As you also know, glycemic control improves dramatically with weight loss. Usually we stop sulfonylurea agents when patients start the program, and, if being used, decrease insulin doses by 33 to 50 percent. Since our specialty is endocrinology, we manage the medications of our patients; if the patient has an endocrinologist, you may want to defer to that individual. Patients need to monitor their blood glucose values at least twice daily on the diet until they are off all medications.
- Cerebral vascular disease: Requires office and patient self-monitoring to diligently avoid hypotension in persons who have a history of stroke or transient ischemic attacks.
- These medications may require special attention:
  - Diuretics: As noted above, may need to be dis-

continued unless the patient has congestive heart failure or significant edema.

- Coumadin: Since intake of vitamin K may increase with consumption of a different diet, prothrombin times may need to be monitored weekly until values are stable.
- Lithium: Changes in diet may require more frequent monitoring of serum lithium and electrolytes by you or the prescribing psychiatrist.
- Trileptal: May cause significant hyponatremia and requires weekly monitoring of the serum sodium values.

- Contact me at askdranderson@aol.com.
- Thank you for empowering your patient to achieve a health-promoting weight.

## EXPANDED GREEN LIGHT CALORIE GUIDE

| FOOD | GREEN<br><br>< 35 CALORIES/ OZ.<br><br>(USE LIBERALLY) | YELLOW<br><br>35–70 CALORIES/ OZ.<br><br>(USE JUDI- CIOUSLY) | RED<br><br>70–110 CALORIES/ OZ.<br><br>(AVOID OR USE SPARINGLY) | RED ALERT<br><br>>110 CALORIES/ OZ.<br><br>(AVOID) |
|---|---|---|---|---|
| **Protein**<br><br>(Include at least two servings of non-fat milk or soy milk and three to four ounces of very lean meat or other protein foods daily) | Non-fat milk, regular or soy, 1 cup**<br><br>Non-fat yogurt, regular or soy, 1 cup*<br><br>Cottage cheese, low-fat, ¾ cup*<br><br>Tofu, 1 cup*<br><br>Egg whites, ¾ cup**<br><br>Egg substitutes, ¾ cup* | Fish, 3 oz.<br><br>Shellfish, 3 oz.*<br><br>Turkey breast w/o skin, 3 oz.*<br><br>Chicken breast w/o skin, 3 oz.*<br><br>Beef, very lean (round, flank, sirloin, tenderloin), 3 oz.<br><br>Pork, very lean (tenderloin and loin chops), 3 oz.<br><br>Vegetarian burger, 3 oz.<br><br>Cottage cheese, ¾ cup | Beef, lean (ground beef and prime grades), 3 oz.<br><br>Pork, lean (shoulder, roast), 3 oz.<br><br>Cheese, low-fat and non-fat, 1 oz. | Pork sausage<br><br>Fried foods<br><br>Hot dogs<br><br>Pizza<br><br>Bacon<br><br>Cheese, regular |
| **Fruits and Vegetables**<br><br>(Include at least five servings of fruits and vegetables daily; see appendices 10.2 and 10.3 for serving sizes) | Fruits, almost all**<br><br>Vegetables, almost all**<br><br>Vegetable soup, 1 cup** | Avocados, ⅓ medium<br><br>Edamame, ½ cup*<br><br>Dried beans and peas, ½ cup*<br><br>Potatoes, ½ cup*<br><br>Sweet potato, ½ cup* | Vegetables, fried, ½ cup | French fries<br><br>Potato chips<br><br>Tortilla chips |

| FOOD | GREEN<br><35<br>CALORIES/<br>OZ.<br>(USE<br>LIBERALLY) | YELLOW<br>35–70<br>CALORIES/<br>OZ.<br>(USE<br>JUDI-<br>CIOUSLY) | RED<br>70–110<br>CALORIES/<br>OZ.<br>(AVOID OR<br>USE<br>SPARINGLY) | RED ALERT<br>>110<br>CALORIES/<br>OZ.<br>(AVOID) |
|---|---|---|---|---|
| **Cereals and Grains**<br>(Include three whole grains daily) | Oatmeal (½ cup cooked)*<br><br>Cereal, high-fiber, dry, most (½–¾ cup) | Pancake, 4-inch, 1<br><br>Whole wheat bread, 1 slice*<br><br>English muffins, ½<br><br>Pasta, whole wheat, ⅓ cup*<br><br>Pasta, ⅓ cup<br><br>Rice, white and brown, ⅓ cup* | Bagel, ½ small<br><br>Bread, white, 1 slice<br><br>Muffin, ½<br><br>Popcorn, plain, air-popped, 3 cups | Crackers<br><br>Granola cereals, most |
| **Fats and Sweets** | Salad dressing, low-calorie, 1 tbsp.<br><br>Butter buds<br><br>Condiments such as ketchup, mustard, and many others<br><br>Low-calorie jelly and jam<br><br>Low-calorie syrup<br><br>Artificial sweeteners | | Angel food cake<br><br>Cookies<br><br>Fruit pies<br><br>Yellow cake | Cake, most<br><br>Candy<br><br>Candy bars<br><br>Nuts, all#<br><br>Margarine<br><br>Butter<br><br>Oils# |

Nutrition Quality Scores: ** excellent; * very good. From Katz[1] and other sources such as calorieking.com and caloriecount.about.com.

# Because of their health benefits, individuals at a healthy body weight can include ¼ cup nuts and very small amounts of olive oil (1–2 teaspoons) daily.

To tell what category a food fits into, divide the calories in a serving of the food by the number of ounces for that serving size, then compare this figure to the calories per ounce in the green, yellow, red, and double red categories. (Serving sizes listed in grams can be converted to ounces by multiplying by 28.4, since 1 ounce = 28.4 grams.)

Appendix 10.2

## Green Light Calorie Guide for
## Weight Loss in the Second Phase*

### APPROXIMATE DAILY SERVINGS OF FOODS FROM THE GREEN AND YELLOW ZONES FOR INDIVIDUALS DESIRING A WEIGHT LOSS OF ONE POUND PER WEEK ON THE SECOND PHASE OF HEALTH AND WEIGHT MANAGEMENT WITH THE SIMPLE DIET

| CURRENT WEIGHT | SERVINGS IN THE GREEN | SERVINGS IN THE YELLOW |
|---|---|---|
| 150 pounds | 6 | 1 |
| 180 pounds | 9 | 2 |
| 210 pounds | 10 | 3 |
| 240 pounds | 12 | 4 |

* The recommended servings of foods in green and yellow categories in this guide for the Second Phase assume continued use of some meal replacements (one entrée and one shake daily).

GREEN LIGHT CALORIE GUIDE FOR WEIGHT
MAINTENANCE APPROXIMATE DAILY SERVINGS OF
FOODS FROM THE GREEN AND YELLOW ZONES FOR
INDIVIDUALS DESIRING TO MAINTAIN THEIR WEIGHT
WITH THE SIMPLE LIFETIME DIET

| CURRENT WEIGHT | SERVINGS IN THE GREEN | SERVINGS IN THE YELLOW |
|---|---|---|
| 150 pounds | 9 | 3 |
| 180 pounds | 10 | 6 |
| 210 pounds | 10 | 8 |
| 240 pounds | 13 | 8 |

- - - - - - - - - - -

## Seven-Day Sample Menu
## for the Simple Lifetime Diet

### 2000 CALORIES PER DAY

| MEAL | DAY 1 | DAY 2 | DAY 3 |
|---|---|---|---|
| **Breakfast** | 1 cup cooked oatmeal<br><br>8 oz. non-fat yogurt<br><br>1 orange | 1 slice whole grain toast<br><br>1 cup non-fat milk<br><br>peach | 1 cup Multigrain Cheerios, 1 cup non-fat milk<br><br>1 cup blueberries |
| **Snack** | 1 cup raw vegetables with non-fat dressing | 1 cup honeydew melon<br><br>1 cup non-fat soy yogurt | 1 cup raw vegetables, ½ cup cherries |
| **Lunch** | 3 oz. tuna on 3 cups mixed greens, with non-fat salad dressing<br><br>1 apple<br><br>1 cup non-fat milk | 1 cup tofu stir fried in non-stick pan with 2 cups mixed red and green pepper, onion, water chestnuts, and celery<br><br>⅓ cup whole grain pasta | 1 cup vegetable bean soup<br><br>1 cup strawberries<br><br>1 cup non-fat yogurt |
| **Snack** | 8 oz. pudding made with 1 cup non-fat milk, ½ cup All Bran cereal | 1 cup raw vegetables | 1 cup watermelon |
| **Dinner** | 3 oz. baked turkey<br><br>½ cup brown rice<br><br>2 cups mixed vegetables (green and red pepper, onion, zucchini) | 3 oz. grilled halibut<br><br>3 cups mixed salad greens with non-fat dressing<br><br>1 cup broccoli<br><br>1 pear | 3 oz. chicken cacciatore<br><br>3 cups mixed green salad<br><br>1 cup carrots |
| **Snack** | 1 cup blackberries | 1 cup cooked oatmeal with 1 cup non-fat soy milk | ½ whole grain English muffin with sugar-free jam, 1 cup non-fat milk |

| MEAL | DAY 4 | DAY 5 | DAY 6 | DAY 7 |
|---|---|---|---|---|
| **Breakfast** | 1 cup non-fat yogurt<br><br>1 cup strawberries<br><br>1 whole wheat English muffin | 1 ½ cups Raisin Bran, 1 cup non-fat soy milk<br><br>½ grapefruit | 1 cup cooked oatmeal, 1 serving raspberry smoothie with 1 cup raspberries and 1 cup non-fat milk | Egg Beater omelet, ½ cup with tomatoes, mushrooms, and green onion<br><br>1 slice whole grain toast<br><br>1 cup cantaloupe |
| **Snack** | 1 cup raspberries | 1 cup raw vegetables | 1 cup mango | 1 cup non-fat yogurt |
| **Lunch** | 1 cup beef stew with trimmed round steak, carrots, celery, tomatoes, onion, pepper, and mushrooms<br><br>1 cup Brussels sprouts<br><br>1 cup non-fat soy milk | 1 cup hearty bean bake with kidney beans, lima beans, tomato, and onion<br><br>1 slice whole grain bread | 3 oz. cubed chicken breast on 3 cups mixed greens and non-fat dressing<br><br>½ cup grapes<br><br>1 cup non-fat soy milk | 3 oz. pork tenderloin<br><br>2 cups summer squash<br><br>1 cup non-fat milk<br><br>1 cup blueberries<br><br>1 cup new red potatoes, boiled |
| **Snack** | 1 cup raw vegetables<br><br>1 cup non-fat soy milk | 1 slice whole grain bread | 1 cup raw vegetables | 1 cup strawberries |
| **Dinner** | 1 cup cooked beans with 1 cup mixed tomatoes, onion, and corn<br><br>1 papaya | 3 oz. lemon-baked tilapia, 1 baked potato<br><br>2 cups green beans<br><br>1 cup cantaloupe | 3 oz. broiled salmon<br><br>2 cups steamed asparagus<br><br>⅓ cup whole grain pasta<br><br>½ cup cooked sweet potatoes | 1 cup lentils with ½ cup barley and 2 cups mixed onion, carrots, potatoes, and tomatoes<br><br>1 slice whole grain bread |
| **Snack** | ½ cup All Bran cereal with 1 cup non-fat milk | 1 cup non-fat soy yogurt with ¾ cup Flax Plus Multigrain cereal<br><br>1 pear | 1 cup sugar-free pudding made with non-fat milk<br><br>1 cup Multigrain Cheerios | 1 cup cooked oatmeal, with 1 cup non-fat milk |

# Notes

1 Gardner, C. D., A. Kiazand, S. Alhassan, S. Kim, R. S. Stafford, R. R. Balise, et al., "Comparison of the Atkins, Zone, Ornish, and LEARN Diets for Change in Weight and Related Risk Factors Among Overweight Premenopausal Women: The A TO Z Weight Loss Study: A Randomized Trial," *The Journal of the American Medical Association* 297 (2007): 969–977.

2 Furlow E. A., J. W. Anderson, "A Systematic Review of Targeted Outcomes Associated with a Medically Supervised Commercial Weight-Loss Program," *Journal of the American Dietetic Association* 109 (2009): 1417–1421.

3 Anderson, J. W., S. B. Conley, A. S. Nicholas, "One Hundred–Pound Weight Losses with an Intensive Behavioral Program: Changes in Risk Factors in 118 Patients with Long-Term Follow-Up," *The American Journal of Clinical Nutrition* 86, no. 2 (2007): 301–307.

4 Anderson, J. W., S. Owen, B. Fajardo, J. Berkson, A. File, S. Cramer, et al., "Assessment of Weight Maintenance at Five Years after Behavioral Weight Loss Intervention," *Obesity* 17, no. 2 (2009): S316. Updated by Sarah Williams, MD, June 2010.

5 Anderson, J. W., S. B. Conley, A. S. Nicholas, "One Hundred–Pound Weight Losses with an Intensive Behavioral Program: Changes in Risk Factors in 118 Patients with Long-Term Follow-Up," *The American Journal of Clinical Nutrition* 86, no. 2 (2007): 301–307.

6 Wang, Y., M. A. Beydoun, L. Liang, B. Caballero, S. K. Kumanyika, "Will All Americans Become Overweight or Obese? Estimating the Progression and Cost of the US Obesity Epidemic," *Obesity* 16, no. 10 (2008): 2323–2330.

7 Knowler, W. C., D. J. Pettitt, P. J. Savage, P. H. Bennett, "Diabetes Incidence in Pima Indians: Contributions of Obesity and Parental Diabetes," *American Journal of Epidemiology* 113 (1981): 144–156.

8 Catenacci, V. A., J. O. Hill, H. R. Wyatt, "The Obesity Epidemic," *Clinics in Chest Medicine* 30, no. 3 (2009): 415–444, vii.

9 Manson, J. E., W. C. Willett, M. J. Stampfer, G. A. Colditz, D. J. Hunter, S. E. Hankinson, et al., "Body Weight and Mortality among Women," *The New England Journal of Medicine* 333, no. 11 (1995): 677–685.

10 Heshka, S., F. Greenway, J. W. Anderson, R. L. Atkinson, J. O. Hill, S. D. Phinney, et al., "Self-Help Weight Loss versus a Structured Commercial Program after 26 Weeks: A Randomized Controlled Study," *The American Journal of Medicine* 109, no. 4 (2000): 282–287.

11 Heymsfield, S. B., C. A. van Mierlo, H. C. van der Knaap, M. Heo, H. I. Frier, "Weight Management Using a Meal Replacement Strategy:

Meta and Pooling Analysis from Six Studies," *International Journal of Obesity and Related Metabolic Disorders* 27, no. 5 (2003): 537–549.

12 Heshka, S., F. Greenway, J. W. Anderson, R. L. Atkinson, J. O. Hill, S. D. Phinney, et al., "Self-Help Weight Loss versus a Structured Commercial Program after 26 Weeks: A Randomized Controlled Study," *The American Journal of Medicine* 109, no. 4 (2000): 282–287.

13 Rock, C. L., B. Pakiz, S. W. Flatt, E. L. Quintana, "Randomized Trial of a Multifaceted Commercial Weight Loss Program," *Obesity* 15, no. 4 (2007): 939–949.

14 Davis, J. M., C. Coleman, J. Kiel, J. Rampolla, T. Hutchisen, L. Ford, et al., "Efficacy of a Meal Replacement Diet Plan Compared to a Food-Based Diet Plan after a Period of Weight Loss and Weight Maintenance: A Randomized Controlled Trial," *Nutrition Journal* 9 (2010): 11–20.

15 Anderson, J. W., L. R. Reynolds, J. Rinsky, H. Bush, C. Washnock, "Effect of a Behavioral and Nutrition Intervention on Weight of Obese Adults: A Randomized, Controlled Clinical Trial," *Postgraduate Medicine* 124, no. 3 (2011).

16 Anderson, J. W., V. Brinkman-Kaplan, C. C. Hamilton, J. E. Logan, R. W. Collins, N. J. Gustafson, "Food-Containing Hypocaloric Diets Are as Effective as Liquid-Supplement Diets for Obese Individuals with NIDDM," *Diabetes Care* 17, no. 6 (1994): 602–604.

17 Anderson, J. W., C. C. Hamilton, E. Crown-Weber, M. Riddlemoser, N. J. Gustafson, "Safety and Effectiveness of a Multidisciplinary Very-Low-Calorie Diet Program for Selected Obese Individuals," *Journal of the American Dietetic Association* 91, no. 12 (1991): 1582–1584.

18 Anderson, J. W., V. L. Brinkman, C. C. Hamilton, "Weight Loss and 2-Y Follow-Up for 80 Morbidly Obese Patients Treated with Intensive Very-Low-Calorie Diet and an Education Program," *The American Journal of Clinical Nutrition* 56 (1992): 244S–246S.

19 Anderson, J. W., V. Brinkman-Kaplan, C. C. Hamilton, J. E. Logan, R. W. Collins, N. J. Gustafson, "Food-Containing Hypocaloric Diets Are as Effective as Liquid-Supplement Diets for Obese Individuals with NIDDM," *Diabetes Care* 17, no. 6 (1994): 602–604.

20 Ibid.

21 Furlow, E. A., J. W. Anderson, "A Systematic Review of Targeted Outcomes Associated with a Medically Supervised Commercial Weight-Loss Program," *Journal of the American Dietetic Association* 109 (2009): 1417–1421.

22 Anderson, J. W., L. Grant, L. Gotthelf, L. T. Stifler, "Weight Loss and Long-Term Follow-Up of Severely Obese Individuals Treated with an Intense Behavioral Program," *International Journal of Obesity* 31, no. 3 (2007): 488–493.

23 Anderson, J. W., S. B. Conley, A. S. Nicholas, "One Hundred–Pound Weight Losses with an Intensive Behavioral Program: Changes in Risk Factors in 118 Patients with Long-Term Follow-Up," *The American Journal of Clinical Nutrition* 86, no. 2 (2007): 301–307.

24 Furlow, E. A., J. W. Anderson, "A Systematic Review of Targeted

Outcomes Associated with a Medically Supervised Commercial Weight-Loss Program," *Journal of the American Dietetic Association* 109 (2009): 1417–1421.

25 Health Management Resources, *The HMR Program for Weight Management: Core Curriculum for Weight Loss Classes* (Boston, MA: Health Management Resources, 2007).

26 Anderson, J.W., M.A. Jhaveri, "Reductions in Medications with Substantial Weight Loss with Behavioral Intervention," *Current Clinical Pharmacology* 5, no. 4 (2010): 232–238.

27 Gardner, C. D., A. Kiazand, S. Alhassan, S. Kim, R. S. Stafford, R. R. Balise, et al., "Comparison of the Atkins, Zone, Ornish, and LEARN Diets for Change in Weight and Related Risk Factors Among Overweight Premenopausal Women: The A TO Z Weight Loss Study: A Randomized Trial," *JAMA* 297 (2007): 969–977.

28 Anderson, J. W., L. R. Reynolds, J. Rinsky, H. Bush, C. Washnock, "Effect of a Behavioral and Nutrition Intervention on Weight of Obese Adults: A Randomized, Controlled Clinical Trial," *Postgraduate Medicine* 124, no. 3 (2011).

29 Blackburn, G. L., "The Low-Fat Imperative," *Obesity* 16, no. 1 (2008): 5–6.

30 Furlow, E. A., J. W. Anderson, "A Systematic Review of Targeted Outcomes Associated with a Medically Supervised Commercial Weight-Loss Program," *Journal of the American Dietetic Association* 109 (2009): 1417–1421.

31 Rock, C. L., B. Pakiz, S. W. Flatt, E. L. Quintana, "Randomized Trial of a Multifaceted Commercial Weight Loss Program," *Obesity* 15, no. 4 (2007): 939–949.

32 Davis, J. M., C. Coleman, J. Kiel, J. Rampolla, T. Hutchisen, L. Ford, et al., "Efficacy of a Meal Replacement Diet Plan Compared to a Food-Based Diet Plan after a Period of Weight Loss and Weight Maintenance: A Randomized Controlled Trial," *Nutrition Journal* 9 (2010): 11–20.

33 Foster, G. D., K. E. Borradaile, S. S. Vander Veur, S. K. Leh, R. J. Dilks, E. M. Goldbacher, et al., "The Effects of a Commercially Available Weight Loss Program among Obese Patients with Type 2 Diabetes: A Randomized Study," *Postgraduate Medicine* 121, no. 5 (2009): 113–118.

34 Anderson, J. W., L. R. Reynolds, J. Rinsky, H. Bush, C. Washnock, "Effect of a Behavioral and Nutrition Intervention on Weight of Obese Adults: A Randomized, Controlled Clinical Trial," *Postgraduate Medicine* 124, no. 3 (September 2011).

35 Furlow, E. A., J. W. Anderson, "A Systematic Review of Targeted Outcomes Associated with a Medically Supervised Commercial Weight-Loss Program," *Journal of the American Dietetic Association* 109 (2009): 1417–1421.

36 Wing, R. R., J. O. Hill, "Successful Weight Loss Maintenance," *Annual Review of Nutrition* 21 (2001): 323–341.

37 Anderson, J.W., M. A. Jhaveri, "Reductions in Medications with Substantial Weight Loss with Behavioral Intervention," *Current Clinical*

*Pharmacology* 5, no. 4 (2010): 232–238.

38 Anderson, J. W., L. R. Reynolds, H. M. Bush, J. L. Rinsky, C. Washnock, "Effect of a Behavioral and Nutrition Intervention on Weight of Obese Adults: A Randomized Controlled, Clinical Trial," in *Postgraduate Medicine* 124, no. 3 (2011).

39 Anderson, J. W., E. C. Konz, "The Use of Very-Low-Calorie Diets (VLCDs) and Meal Replacement Use for Weight Control," in *Food, Diet and Obesity*, ed. D. Mela (Cambridge, UK: Woodhead Publishing, 2005), 379–411.

40 Health Management Resources, *Follow-up Training #2010A* (Boston, MA: Health Management Resources, 2010).

41 Katz, D.L., V. Y. Njike, L. Q. Rhee, A. Reingold, K. T. Ayoob, "Performance Characteristics of NuVal and the Overall Nutrition Quality Index (ONQI)," *The American Journal of Clinical Nutrition*, 91 (Suppl) (2010): 1102S–1108S.

42 Anderson, J. W., S. Owen, B. Fajardo, J. Berkson, A. File, S. Cramer S., et al., "Assessment of Weight Maintenance at Five Years after Behavioral Weight Loss Intervention," *Obesity* 17, no. 2 (2009): S316. Updated by Sarah Williams, MD, June 2010.

43 Anderson, J. W., S. B. Conley, A. S. Nicholas, "One Hundred–Pound Weight Losses with an Intensive Behavioral Program: Changes in Risk Factors in 118 Patients with Long-Term Follow-Up," *The American Journal of Clinical Nutrition* 86, no. 2 (2007): 301–307.

44 Blackburn, G. L., D. Rothacker, "Ten-Year Self-Management of Weight Using a Meal Replacement Diet Plan: Comparison with Matched Controls," *Obesity Research* 11 (2003): A103.

45 Sjostrom, L., K. Narbro, C. D. Sjostrom, K. Karason, B. Larsson, H. Wedel, et al., "Effects of Bariatric Surgery on Mortality in Swedish Obese Subjects," *The New England Journal of Medicine* 357, no. 8 (2007): 741–752.

46 Omalu, B. I., D. G. Ives, A. M. Buhari, J. L. Lindner, P. R. Schauer, C. H. Wecht, et al., "Death Rates and Causes of Death after Bariatric Surgery for Pennsylvania Residents, 1995 to 2004," *Archives of Surgery* 142, no. 10 (2007): 923–928.

47 Flum, D. R., L. Salem, J. A. Elrod, E. P. Dellinger, A. Cheadle, L. Chan, "Early Mortality among Medicare Beneficiaries Undergoing Bariatric Surgical Procedures," *The Journal of the American Medical Association* 294, no. 15 (2005): 1903–1908.

48 Encinosa, W. E., D. M. Bernard, C. C. Chen, C. A. Steiner, "Healthcare Utilization and Outcomes after Bariatric Surgery," *Medical Care* 44 (2006): 706–712.

49 Sjostrom, L., K. Narbro, C. D. Sjostrom, K. Karason, B. Larsson, H. Wedel, et al., "Effects of Bariatric Surgery on Mortality in Swedish Obese Subjects," *The New England Journal of Medicine* 357, no. 8 (2007): 741–752.

50 Phillips, E., J. Ponce, S. A. Cunneen, S. Bhoyrul, E. Gomez, S. Ikramuddin, et al., "Safety and Effectiveness of Realize Adjustable Gastric Band: 3-year Prospective Study in the United States," *Surgery for Obesity and Related Diseases* 5, no. 5 (2009): 588–597.

51 Mittermair, R. P., S. Obermuller, A. Perathoner, M. Sieb, F. Aigner, R. Margreiter, "Results and Complications after Swedish Adjustable Gastric Banding—10 Years Experience," *Obesity Surgery* 19, no. 12 (2009): 1636–1641.

52 Anderson, J. W., S. B. Conley, A. S. Nicholas, "One Hundred–Pound Weight Losses with an Intensive Behavioral Program: Changes in Risk Factors in 118 Patients with Long-Term Follow-Up," *The American Journal of Clinical Nutrition* 86, no. 2 (2007): 301–307.

53 Hu, F. B, W. C. Willett, "Optimal Diets for Prevention of Coronary Heart Disease," *The Journal of the American Medical Association* 288, no. 20 (2002): 2569–2578.

54 Anderson, J. W., "Lifestyle Medicine for the 21st Century: Reversing Diabesity" (lecture, Feather River Hospital, Paradise, CA, October 2, 2008).

55 Anderson, J.W., M. A. Jhaveri, "Reductions in Medications with Substantial Weight Loss with Behavioral Intervention," *Current Clinical Pharmacology* 5 (2010): 232–238.

56 Manson, J. E., et al., "Walking Compared with Vigorous Exercise for the Prevention of Cardiovascular Events in Women," *The New England Journal of Medicine* 347, no. 10 (2002): 716–725.

57 Taylor, J. B., *My Stroke of Insight: A Brain Scientist's Personal Journey* (New York: Penguin Books, Ltd., 2010).

58 Helmstetter, S., and B. Schwartz, *Self-talk for Weight Loss* (New York: St. Martin's Press, 1996).

59 Furlow, E. A., J. W. Anderson, "A Systematic Review of Targeted Outcomes Associated with a Medically Supervised Commercial Weight-Loss Program," *Journal of the American Dietetic Association* 109 (2009): 1417–1421.

# Bibliography

Alinia, S., O. Heis, I. Tetens, "The Potential Association Between Fruit Intake and Body Weight—a Review," *Obesity Reviews* 10 (2010): 639–647.

Anderson, J. W., *Diabetes: A Practical New Guide to Healthy Living* (London, United Kingdom: Martin Dunitz, Ltd., 1981), 1–293.

Anderson, J. W., "Weight Loss and Lipid Changes with Low-Energy Diets," *Agro Food* 18, no. 5 (2007): 1–2.

Anderson, J. W., "Whole-Grains Intake and Risk for Coronary Heart Disease," in *Whole-Grain Foods in Health and Disease*, ed. L. Marquart, J. L. Slavin, and G. Fulcher (St. Paul, MN: American Association of Cereal Chemists, 2002), 100–114.

Anderson, J. W., et al., "Food-Containing Hypocaloric Diets Are as Effective as Liquid-Supplement Diets for Obese Individuals with NIDDM," *Diabetes Care* 17, no. 6 (1994): 602–604.

Anderson, J. W., et al., "Health Benefits of Dietary Fiber," *Nutrition Reviews* 67, no. 4 (2009): 188–205.

Anderson, J. W., et al., "Long-Term Weight-Loss Maintenance: A Meta-Analysis of US Studies," *The American Journal of Clinical Nutrition* 74, no. 5 (2001): 579–584.

Anderson, J. W., et al., "Long-Term Weight Maintenance After an Intensive Weight-Loss Program," *Journal of the American College of Nutrition* 18, no. 6 (1999): 620–627.

Anderson, J. W., et al., "Safety and Effectiveness of a Multidisciplinary Very-Low-Calorie Diet Program for Selected Obese Individuals," *Journal of the American Dietetic Association* 91, no. 12 (1991): 1582–1584.

Anderson, J. W., et al., "Soy Compared to Casein Meal Replacement Shakes with Energy-Restricted Diets for Obese Women: Randomized Controlled Trial," *Metabolism* 56, no. 2 (2007): 280–288.

Anderson, J. W., et al., "Weight Loss and Long-Term Follow-Up of Severely Obese Individuals Treated with an Intense Behavioral Program," *International Journal of Obesity* 31, no. 3 (2007): 488–493.

Anderson, J. W., M. M. Breecher, *Dr. Anderson's Antioxidant, Antiaging Health Program* (New York, NY: Carroll & Graf, 1996), 1–270.

Anderson, J. W., V. L. Brinkman, C. C. Hamilton, "Weight Loss and 2-Y Follow-Up for 80 Morbidly Obese Patients Treated with Intensive Very-Low-Calorie Diet and an Education Program," *The American Journal of Clinical Nutrition* 56, no. 1 (1992): 244S–246S.

Anderson, J. W., S. B. Conley, A. S. Nicholas, "One Hundred–Pound Weight Losses with an Intensive Behavioral Program: Changes in Risk Factors in 118 Patients with Long-Term Follow-Up," *The American Journal of Clinical Nutrition* 86, no. 2 (2007): 301–307.

Anderson, J. W., N. J. Gustafson, *Dr. Anderson's High-Fiber Fitness Plan* (Lexington, KY: The University Press of Kentucky, 1994).

Anderson, J. W., C. C. Hamilton, V. Brinkman-Kaplan, "Benefits and Risks of an Intensive Very-Low-Calorie Diet Program for Severe Obesity," *The American Journal of Gastroenterology* 87, no. 1 (1992): 6–15.

Anderson, J. W., L. H. Hoie, "Weight Loss and Lipid Changes with Low-Energy Diets: Comparator Study of Milk-Based Versus Soy-Based Liquid Meal Replacement Interventions," *Journal of the American College of Nutrition* 24, no. 3 (2005): 210–216.

Anderson, J. W., M. A. Jhaveri, "Reductions in Medications with Substantial Weight Loss with Behavioral Intervention," *Current Clinical Pharmacology* 5, no. 4 (2010): 232–238.

Anderson, J. W., C. W. Kendall, D. J. Jenkins, "Importance of Weight Management in Type 2 Diabetes: Review with Meta-Analysis of Clinical Studies," *Journal of the American College of Nutrition* 22, no. 5 (2003): 331–339.

Anderson, J. W., E. C. Konz, "The Use of Very-Low-Calorie Diets (VLCDs) and Meal Replacement Use for Weight Control," in *Food, Diet and Obesity*, ed. D. Mela (Cambridge, UK: Woodhead Publishing, 2005), 379–411.

Anderson, J. W., E. C. Konz, D. J. Jenkins, "Health Advantages and Disadvantages of Weight-Reducing Diets: A Computer Analysis and Critical Review," *Journal of the American College of Nutrition* 19, no. 5 (2000): 578–590.

Anderson, J. W., C. Liu, R. J. Kryscio, "Blood Pressure Response to Transcendental Meditation: A Meta-Analysis," *American Journal of Hypertension* 21, no. 3 (2008): 310–316.

Anderson, J. W., S. Owen, B. Fajardo, J. Berkson, A. File, S. Cramer, L. Gotthelf, "Assessment of Weight Maintenance at Five Years after Behavioral Weight Loss Intervention," *Obesity* 17, no. 2 (2009): S316. Updated by Sarah Williams, MD, June 2010.

Anderson, J. W., L. R. Reynolds, H. M. Bush, J. L. Rinsky, C. Washnock, "Effect of a Behavioral and Nutrition Intervention on Weight of Obese Adults: A Randomized Controlled, Clinical Trial," in *Postgraduate Medicine* 124, no. 3 (2011).

Anderson, J. W., B. Sieling, "High Fiber Diets for Obese Diabetic Patients," *Obesity & Bariatric Medicine* 9, no. 109 (1980): 113.

Blackburn, G. L., "The Low-Fat Imperative," *Obesity* 16, no. 1 (2008): 5–6.

Blackburn, G. L., D. Rothacker, "Ten-Year Self-Management of Weight Using a Meal Replacement Diet Plan: Comparison with Matched Controls," *Obesity Research* 11 (2003): A103.

Bouchard, C., "Childhood Obesity: Are Genetic Differences Involved?"

*The American Journal of Clinical Nutrition* 89, no. 5 (2009): 1494S–1501S.

Buijsse, B., et al., "Fruit and Vegetable Intakes and Subsequent Changes in Body Weight in European Populations: Results From the Project on Diet, Obesity, and Genes (DiOGenes)," *The American Journal of Clinical Nutrition* 90, no. 1 (2009): 202–209.

Butryn, M. L., et al., "Consistent Self-Monitoring of Weight: A Key Component of Successful Weight Loss Maintenance," *Obesity* 15, no. 12 (2007): 3091–3096.

Catenacci, V. A., et al., "Physical Activity Patterns in the National Weight Control Registry," *Obesity* 16, no. 1 (2008): 153–161.

Catenacci, V. A., J. O. Hill, H. R. Wyatt, "The Obesity Epidemic," *Clinics in Chest Medicine* 30, no. 3 (2009): 415–444, vii.

Davis, L. M., et al., "Efficacy of a Meal Replacement Diet Plan Compared to a Food-Based Diet Plan after a Period of Weight Loss and Weight Maintenance: A Randomized Controlled Trial," *Nutrition Journal* 9 (2010): 11–20.

Dennis, E. A., et al., "Water Consumption Increases Weight Loss During a Hypocaloric Diet Intervention in Middle-Aged and Older Adults," *Obesity* 18, no. 2 (2010): 300–307.

Deslandes, A., et al., "Exercise and Mental Health: Many Reasons to Move," *Neuropsychobiology* 59, no. 4 (2009): 191–198.

Elfhag, K., S. Rossner, "Who Succeeds in Maintaining Weight Loss? A Conceptual Review of Factors Associated with Weight Loss Maintenance and Weight Regain," *Obesity Reviews* 6 (2005): 67–85.

Esselstyn Jr., C. B., "Resolving the Coronary Artery Disease Epidemic Through Plant-Based Nutrition," *Preventive Cardiology* 4, no. 4 (2001): 171–177.

Flechtner-Mors, M., et al., "Metabolic and Weight Loss Effects of Long-Term Dietary Intervention in Obese Patients: Four-Year Results," *Obesity Research* 8 (2000): 399–402.

Flegal, K. M., et al., "Prevalence and Trends in Obesity Among US Adults, 1999–2008," *The Journal of the American Medical Association* 303, no. 3 (2010): 235–241.

Flint, A. J., et al., "Excess Weight and the Risk of Incident Coronary Heart Disease Among Men and Women," *Obesity* 18, no. 2 (2010): 377–383.

Fogelhorn, M., et al., "Effects of Walking Training on Weight Maintenance After a Very-Low-Energy Diet in Premenopausal Obese Women," *Archives of Internal Medicine* 160 (2000): 2177–2184.

Fogelhorn, M., K. Kukkonen-Harjula, "Does Physical Activity Prevent Weight Gain—A Systematic Review," *Obesity Reviews* 1 (2000): 95–111.

Foster, G. D., et al., "The Effects of a Commercially Available Weight Loss Program among Obese Patients with Type 2 Diabetes: A Randomized Study," *Postgraduate Medicine* 121, no. 5 (2009): 113–118.

Furlow, E. A., J. W. Anderson, "A Systematic Review of Targeted Outcomes Associated with a Medically Supervised Commercial Weight-

Loss Program," *Journal of the American Dietetic Association* 109 (2009): 1417–1421.

Gardner, C. D., et al., "Comparison of the Atkins, Zone, Ornish, and LEARN Diets for Change in Weight and Related Risk Factors Among Overweight Premenopausal Women: The A TO Z Weight Loss Study. A Randomized Trial," *The Journal of the American Medical Association* 297 (2007): 969–977.

Heber, D., S. Bowerman, *What Color Is Your Diet?* (New York: Harper-Collins, 2001), 1–300.

Herring, M. P., P. J. O'Connor, R. K. Dishman, "The Effect of Exercise Training on Anxiety Symptoms Among Patients: A Systematic Review," *Archives of Internal Medicine* 170, no. 4 (2010): 321–331.

Heshka, S., et al., "Self-Help Weight Loss versus a Structured Commercial Program after 26 Weeks: A Randomized Controlled Study," *The American Journal of Medicine* 109, no. 4 (2000): 282–287.

Heshka, S., et al., "Weight Loss with Self-Help Compared with a Structured Commercial Program: A Randomized Trial," *The Journal of the American Medical Association* 289, no. 14 (2003): 1792–1798.

Heymsfield, S. B., et al., "Weight Management Using a Meal Replacement Strategy: Meta and Pooling Analysis from Six Studies," *International Journal of Obesity and Related Metabolic Disorders* 27, no. 5 (2003): 537–549.

Hu, F. B., W. C. Willett, "Optimal Diets for Prevention of Coronary Heart Disease," *The Journal of the American Medical Association* 288, no. 20 (2002): 2569–2578.

Jakicic, J. M., "The Effect of Physical Activity on Body Weight," *Obesity* 17 (2010): S34–S38.

Jhaveri, M. A., J. W. Anderson, "Sequential Changes of Serum Amino-transferase Levels in Severely Obese Patients After Losing Weight Through Enrollment in a Behavioral Weight Loss Program," *Postgraduate Medicine* 122, no. 4 (2010): 206–212.

Katz, D. L., et al., "Performance Characteristics of NuVal and the Overall Nutritional Quality Index (ONQI)," *The American Journal of Clinical Nutrition* 91, no. 4 (2010): 1102S–1108S.

Kiehm, T. G., J. W. Anderson, and K. Ward, "Beneficial Effects of a High Carbohydrate, High Fiber Diet on Hyperglycemic Diabetic Men," *The American Journal of Clinical Nutrition* 29 (1976): 895–899.

Kiernan, M. et al., "Men Gain Additional Psychological Benefits by Adding Exercise to a Weight-Loss Program," *Obesity Research* 9 (2001): 770–777.

Knowler, W. C., et al., "Diabetes Incidence in Pima Indians: Contributions of Obesity and Parental Diabetes," *American Journal of Epidemiology* 113 (1981): 144–156.

Kuller, L. H., "Cardiovascular Disease Is Preventable Among Women," *Expert Review of Cardiovascular Therapy* 8, no. 2 (2010): 175–187.

Larson, E. B., et al., "Exercise Is Associated with Reduced Risk for Incident Dementia Among Persons 65 Years of Age and Older," *Annals of Internal Medicine* 144, no. 2 (2006): 73–81.

Lee, Y., J. Kim, J. H. Back, "The Influence of Multiple Lifestyle Behaviors on Cognitive Function in Older Persons Living in the Community," *Preventive Medicine* 48, no. 1 (2009): 86–90.

Ma, J., and L. Xiao, "Obesity and Depression in US Women: Results from the 2005–2006 National Health and Nutritional Examination Survey," *Obesity* 18, no. 2 (2010): 347–353.

Major, A., and J. Anderson, "An Adolescent Weight Reduction Program Including Meal Replacements and Parental Involvement Decreases Body Weight and Fat Mass of Obese Adolescents," *Obesity Research* 12 (2004): A16.

Manson, J. E., et al., "Body Weight and Mortality among Women," *The New England Journal of Medicine* 333, no. 11 (1995): 677–685.

Manson, J. E., et al., "Walking Compared with Vigorous Exercise for the Prevention of Cardiovascular Events in Women," *The New England Journal of Medicine* 347, no. 10 (2002): 716–725.

McTiernan, A., et al., "Exercise Effect on Weight and Body Fat in Men and Women," *Obesity* 15, no. 6 (2007): 1496–1512.

Mittermair, R. P., S. Obermuller, A. Perathoner, M. Sieb, F. Aigner, R. Margreiter, "Results and Complications after Swedish Adjustable Gastric Banding—10 Years Experience," *Obesity Surgery* 19, no. 12 (2009): 1636–1641.

Myers, J., et al., "Exercise Capacity and Mortality Among Men Referred for Exercise Testing," *The New England Journal of Medicine* 346, no. 11 (2002): 793–801.

Nutrition and Allergies NDA EFSA Panel on Dietetic Products, "Scientific Opinion on the Substantiation of Health Claims Related to Meal Replacements for Weight Control . . . and Reduction in Body Weight . . . and Maintenance of Body Weight After Weight Loss . . . ," *EFSA Journal* 8, no. 2 (2010): 1466–1485.

Omalu, B. I., D. G. Ives, A. M. Buhari, J. L. Lindner, P. R. Schauer, C. H. Wecht, et al., "Death Rates and Causes of Death after Bariatric Surgery for Pennsylvania Residents, 1995 to 2004," *Archives of Surgery* 142, no. 10 (2007): 923–928.

Ornish, D., et al., "Can Lifestyle Changes Reverse Coronary Heart Disease? The Lifestyle Heart Trial," *Lancet* 336 (1990): 129–133.

Pasupuleti, V. K., J. W. Anderson, *Nutraceuticals, Glycemic Health and Type 2 Diabetes* (Ames, IA: Blackwell Publishing Professional, 2008), 1–489.

Phillips, E., J. Ponce, S. A. Cunneen, S. Bhoyrul, E. Gomez, S. Ikramuddin, et al., "Safety and Effectiveness of Realize Adjustable Gastric Band: 3-year Prospective Study in the United States," *Surgery for Obesity and Related Diseases* 5, no. 5 (2009): 588–597.

Pouwer, F., N. Kupper, M. C. Adriaanse, "Does Emotional Stress Cause Type 2 Diabetes Mellitus? A Review from the European Depression in Diabetes (EDID) Research Consortium," *Discovery Medicine* 9, no. 45 (2010): 112–118.

Puhl, R. M., C. A. Heuer, "The Stigma of Obesity: A Review and Update," *Obesity* 17, no. 5 (2009): 941–964.

Racette, S. B., et al., "Exercise Enhances Dietary Compliance During Moderate Energy Restriction in Obese Women," *The American Journal of Clinical Nutrition* 62 (2001): 345–349.

Raynor, D. A., et al., "Television Viewing and Long-Term Weight Maintenance: Results From the National Weight Control Registry," *Obesity* 14, no. 10 (2006): 1816–1824.

Reynolds, L. R., J. W. Anderson, "Practical Office Strategies for Weight Management of the Obese Diabetic Individual," *Endocrine Practice* 10, no. 2 (2004): 153–159.

Rock, C. L., et al., "Randomized Trial of a Multifaceted Commercial Weight Loss Program," *Obesity* 15, no. 4 (2007): 939–949.

Rolls, B. J., L. S. Roe, J. S. Meengs, "Portion Size Can Be Used Strategically to Increase Vegetable Consumption in Adults," *The American Journal of Clinical Nutrition* 91, no. 4 (2010): 913–922.

Rolls, B. J., L. S. Roe, J. S. Meengs, "Reductions in Portion Size and Energy Density of Foods Are Additive and Lead to Sustained Decreases in Energy Intake," *The American Journal of Clinical Nutrition* 83, no. 1 (2006): 11–17.

Schmidt, W. D., C. J. Biwer, L. K. Kalscheuer, "Effects of Long Versus Short Bout Exercise on Fitness and Weight Loss in Overweight Females," *Journal of the American College of Nutrition* 20, no. 5 (2001): 494–501.

Schneider, R. H., et al., "Long-Term Effects of Stress Reduction on Mortality in Persons ≥ 55 Years of Age with Systemic Hypertension," *The American Journal of Cardiology* 95, no. 9 (2005): 1060–1064.

Sjostrom, L., K. Narbro, C. D. Sjostrom, K. Karason, B. Larsson, H. Wedel, et al., "Effects of Bariatric Surgery on Mortality in Swedish Obese Subjects," *The New England Journal of Medicine* 357, no. 8 (2007): 741–752.

Snowdon, D. A., "Aging and Alzheimer's Disease: Lessons from the Nun Study," *Gerontologist* 37, no. 2 (1997): 150–156.

Wadden, T. A., M. L. Butryn, C. Wilson, "Lifestyle Modification for the Management of Obesity," *Gastroenterology* 132, no. 6 (2007): 2226–2238.

Wang, Y., et al., "Will All Americans Become Overweight or Obese? Estimating the Progression and Cost of the US Obesity Epidemic," *Obesity* 16, no. 10 (2008): 2323–2330.

Wing, R. R., and J. O. Hill, "Successful Weight Loss Maintenance," *Annual Review of Nutrition* 21 (2001): 323–341.

Wyatt, H. R., et al., "Long-Term Weight Loss and Breakfast in Subjects in the National Weight Control Registry," *Obesity Research* 10, no. 2 (2002): 78–82.

Wyatt, H. R., et al., "Resting Energy Expenditure in Reduced-Obese Subjects in the National Weight Control Registry," *The American Journal of Clinical Nutrition* 69, no. 6 (1999): 1189–1193.

# Index

Page numbers in **bold** indicate charts or tables; those in *italics* indicate illustrations.